The Natural Mind

Books by Andrew Weil, M.D.

THE NATURAL MIND
A Revolutionary Approach to the Drug Problem

THE MARRIAGE OF THE SUN AND MOON
Dispatches from the Frontiers of Consciousness

FROM CHOCOLATE TO MORPHINE
Everything You Need to Know About
Mind-Altering Drugs (with Winifred Rosen)

HEALTH AND HEALING
The Philosophy of Integrative Medicine
and Optimum Health

NATURAL HEALTH, NATURAL MEDICINE
The Complete Guide to Wellness and Self-Care
for Optimum Health

SPONTANEOUS HEALING
How to Discover and Enhance the Body's
Ability to Maintain and Heal Itself

EIGHT WEEKS TO OPTIMUM HEALTH
A Proven Program for Taking Full Advantage
of Your Body's Natural Healing Power

EATING WELL FOR OPTIMUM HEALTH
The Essential Guide to Food, Diet, and Nutrition

THE HEALTHY KITCHEN
Recipes for a Better Body, Mind, and Spirit
(with Rosie Daley)

HEALTHY AGING
A Lifelong Guide to Your Physical and
Spiritual Well-Being

The Natural Mind

A Revolutionary Approach
to the Drug Problem

Andrew Weil

Revised Edition

HOUGHTON MIFFLIN COMPANY
BOSTON · NEW YORK

For information about permission to reproduce selections from this book,
write to trade.permissions@hmhco.com or to Permissions, Houghton Mifflin
Harcourt Publishing Company, 3 Park Avenue, 19th Floor, New York, New
York 10016.

Visit our Web site: www.hmhco.com

Library of Congress Cataloging-in-Publication Data
Weil, Andrew.
The natural mind : a revolutionary approach to
the drug problem / Andrew Weil. — Rev. ed.
p. cm.
Includes bibliographical references and index.
ISBN 0-618-46513-8
ISBN 978-0-618-46513-2
1. Psychotropic drugs. 2. Consciousness.
3. Altered states of consciousness. I. Title.
BF207.W45 2004 154.4—dc22 2004054061

Printed in the United States of America

Book design by Robert Overholtzer

DOH 10 9 8
4500601528

Contents

Preface to the 2004 Edition   vii

Preface to the 1998 Edition   ix

Preface to the 1985 Edition   xi

1. What This Book Is About   1

2. Why People Take Drugs   14

3. Is Anything Wrong with It?   33

4. What No One Wants to Know About Marijuana   63

5. Clues from the Amazon   85

6. The Solar Mind: Straight Thinking   101

7. A Trip to the Moon: Deep Thinking   129

8. The Only Solution to the Drug Problem   163

9. Where to Go from Here   174

   Acknowledgments   179

   Afterword   181

   Works Cited   187

   Suggested Reading   191

   Index   193

Preface to the 2004 Edition

FOR THE FIRST TIME since its original publication in 1972 I have decided to make significant revisions in the text of *The Natural Mind*. My reason for doing so is simply to eliminate language and references that would sound dated to today's readers.

Principally, I have changed the term "stoned thinking" that was recurrent in chapters 7, 8, and 9 of previous editions. In contemporary culture "stoned" now exclusively denotes "under the influence of marijuana," which directly undercuts my intended meaning. A major point of this book is that highs can be had without drugs because they are states of consciousness that arise from within us. From the vantage point of a new century I can see that the name I used for the useful kind of thinking that can occur in high states was not the right choice. It has also allowed my critics to contend that I am, in fact, promoting drug use. ("Everybody must get stoned.") I am not. What I am promoting in these pages and in all my subsequent work is a new way of thinking.

Readers who know my second book, *The Marriage of the Sun and Moon: Dispatches from the Frontiers of Consciousness*, will recognize the terms "solar mind" and "lunar mind" that I have introduced to this work. I have kept "straight thinking" for the operations of the solar mind, because it is accurate, but I will now use "deep thinking" for its lunar counterpart. And I want readers to understand that I value and use both types of thinking in my own life and work, because both have their place and particular application.

I have tried to make the style and language of the book more contemporary, but I have not changed any of its messages. The inability of our society to make progress with the drug problem is astonishing and frustrating. The drug problem is much worse now than it was when *The Natural Mind* first appeared more than thirty years ago — small wonder, since all attempts to deal with it are still based in straight thinking.

ANDREW WEIL

Vail, Arizona
January 2004

Preface to the 1998 Edition

IT'S A GREAT SOURCE of satisfaction that *The Natural Mind*, my first book, originally published in 1972, is still used in college courses on drugs and drug policy and continues to exert influence on how people think about psychoactive drugs and altered states of consciousness. I am also dismayed that our society still clings to useless notions about drug use, imagining that it can solve the drug problem by trying to make disliked drugs and their users go away.

In recent years, my professional work has focused on health and healing, and in particular, on the development of new educational models for the training of physicians. When I am interviewed by the media on these subjects, reporters frequently ask pointed questions about my earlier work, thinking that I might wish to disown *The Natural Mind* and the two books that followed it. Far from it. The philosophy of my first book is the same philosophy that underlies my writing about health. Just as *The Natural Mind* argues that highs originate within the human nervous system and are elicited or triggered by drugs, so my later works propose that healing responses originate within us and can be elicited or triggered by the treatments applied. In fact, the seed of my thinking about conventional and alternative medicine can be found in chapter 7 of this book.

At this remove, *The Natural Mind* seems like an old friend. I am very pleased to see it out in this new edition.

Tucson, Arizona
January 1998

Preface to the 1985 Edition

READING OVER this book in order to bring it up to date left me feeling that I should explain its tone. To do so I must describe the circumstances of its creation.

The Natural Mind is a product of the sixties. It grew out of experiences I had in college and medical school in Boston from 1960 through 1968 and during a medical internship in San Francisco the following year, when streets and campuses were battle zones. Though written in 1971 and first published in 1972, the book embodies the spirit of the preceding decade and the generation that came of age in it, full of optimism, righteous anger, and openness to change.

Just before I started writing I spent a frustrating year working at the National Institute of Mental Health in a suburb of Washington, D.C. I was serving military time in the Public Health Service, wanting only to avoid political confrontations. This was 1969, however, the first year of Richard Nixon's presidency, when social turmoil and polarization were increasing daily. The National Institute of Mental Health was caught up in the storm, and despite my best intentions, so was I. My administrative superiors came to regard me as a political liability. They opened my mail, tried to prevent legislators and reporters from reaching me, and threatened to send me to Vietnam if I did not behave.

The problem was marijuana, then as now a red-hot issue because of its countercultural symbolism and associations with "undesirable" elements of society. I had designed and carried out laboratory studies of marijuana with human volunteers — some of the first research of its kind — in my senior year of medical school. The results were published in leading journals in 1968 and 1969 and got a great deal of publicity, including front-page coverage in the *New York Times*.

I had also used marijuana myself in order to know its effects firsthand. The conclusions I came to about it were sound, but they did not support the establishment view of the drug as an unmitigated threat to mental health, more menacing than alcohol. I published my findings in the naive belief that honest information on the subject would help resolve the acrimonious debate that was tearing families and communities apart. For the first time in my life I found that telling the truth got me in trouble. My employers did not want the public to know what I had discovered about marijuana, and they resented all the attention my published work continued to receive.

By the end of the first half of what was to have been a two-year stint as a federal employee and commissioned officer, my working life in Washington had become intolerable. I was typed as a rebel and troublemaker, was barred from doing any work related to marijuana or other drugs, then was ordered to move to the federal addiction hospital in Lexington, Kentucky, to work as a ward doctor for heroin addicts. I refused to go. Eventually, I resigned the job and commission and was denied military credit for the year I had served. I applied for deferment as a conscientious objector, but stated that I would not do any alternative service for a system that seemed to me committed to dishonesty.

My first act as an unemployed ex-official of the U.S. government was to go off to an Indian reservation in South Dakota to study with a Lakota medicine man, Leonard Crowdog. I wanted to learn from him about herbal medicine and about ways of changing consciousness without drugs. On the reservation I participated in sweat lodge ceremonies, grew a beard, and "dropped out." When I returned to my house in rural northern Virginia, I found my draft board had granted me conscientious objector status without a hearing. Suddenly and unexpectedly, I had no obligations and nothing but free time. Over the next year (1970–71), I started to practice yoga, experiment with vegetarianism, and learn to meditate. I also reflected on events of the recent past and began to write.

What I wrote was the original edition of this book, now in its second decade in print. The context of the writing influenced its tone, which flashes anger in spots and delights in sniping at such institutions as universities, professional medicine and psychiatry, and, of course, the National Institute of Mental Health. I have not altered tone or style in preparing this edition. I have made a number of textual changes in the interest of accuracy, reflecting what I have learned since 1971.

If the book's style now seems to require explanation, I am gratified that the content withstands the test of time, even though much has happened in the interim with regard to drugs and consciousness. No one in 1971 foresaw the epidemic of cocaine use that now prevails, for example, or understood cigarette addiction to be the hardest of all drug addictions to break and our most serious public health problem. Few people believed that alternative medical treatments would become as popular as they are now, or that scientific study of body-mind interactions would ever become respectable. No one knew about endorphins, the morphine-like molecules made in every human brain that serve as our own internal narcotics. None of these changes and discoveries are inconsistent with the ideas in the book; in fact, all follow logically from them.

At the time of its first publication *The Natural Mind* drew much praise for its original and radical insights. It also drew harsh condemnation from a few prominent critics within the medical establishment who saw it as an apology for drug use. They misread my arguments and attacked me for saying that human beings are born with a need to use drugs. What I wrote was that human beings are born with a drive to experiment with ways of changing consciousness. Drugs are but one of many possible techniques, having their own risks and limitations. The idea that it is normal to seek changes in consciousness has never been discredited.

The Natural Mind argues that high states originate within the human nervous system rather than in any external substances. Research on endorphins and other neurochemicals strongly supports this theory. The book also insists that such states have great positive potential, a suggestion confirmed by demonstrations of the power of the mind, when not in its ordinary mode, to modify functions of the body and counteract disease. I have developed and explored that theme through the intervening years in my own investigations and writing. My later books — *The Marriage of the Sun and Moon* (1980), *From Chocolate to Morphine* (1983), and, especially, *Health and Healing* (1984) — all expand on it.

Over the years I have received many comments from readers of *The Natural Mind*. Most frequently, readers tell me that the book articulates ideas they have had and makes them feel better about themselves, specifically about their interest in experiencing other forms of consciousness, which they had learned to regard as abnormal and unhealthy. These comments reveal the burden imposed on individuals by our culture in its failure to come to terms with the human need for variations in conscious experience.

If I were to write *The Natural Mind* today, it would be much shorter. I would omit a lot of the argument and focus on the new way of thinking that is the heart of the book: The root of the drug problem is the failure of our culture to provide for a basic human need. Once we recognize the importance and value of other states of consciousness, we can begin to teach people, particularly the young, how to satisfy their needs without drugs. The chief advantage of drugs is that they are quick and effective, producing desired results without requiring effort. Their chief disadvantage is that they fail us over time; used regularly and frequently, they do not maintain the experiences sought and, instead, limit our options and freedom.

What I mean by the "new way of thinking" in the book concerns conceptual models. I believe that we cannot know reality directly through intellectual activity. Instead, we construct models or paradigms of reality through which we interpret and make sense of our experience. There is much talk these days of "paradigm shifts" and conflicts between proponents of alternative models in many fields of human activity, from physics to medicine to the social sciences. Alternative models are neither right nor wrong, just more or less useful in allowing us to operate well in the world and discover more and better options for solving problems.

The Natural Mind suggests a new model for solving the drug problem and other problems like it, all of which will continue to worsen until we change old conceptions. The new model I propose postulates that consciousness is central and primary. This reversal of the prevailing scientific view (which sees consciousness as secondary and peripheral to material reality) changes conventional ideas of cause-and-effect relationships. Furthermore, the new model substitutes "both/and" formulations for the "either/or" formulations of the old model, opening more possibilities for personal freedom, reducing the discomfort of existence, and making life much more creative.

That is the essence of *The Natural Mind*. Its message is as timely now as when it first appeared, since the need to rethink basic conceptions about drugs and consciousness is as urgent now as ever.

Tucson, Arizona
May 1985

The Natural Mind

1. What This Book Is About

THIS BOOK IS AN EXPOSITION of a theory that can help us. It is not a primer of pharmacology or a program for social reform. Rather, it is the germ of a new way of thinking about drugs and consciousness — a way that creates possibilities for solving a problem that divides us bitterly in our nation, in our schools, and in our homes.

I have been actively interested in drugs that affect the mind for the past ten years, and during that time I have had many opportunities to write this book. I have declined to do so until now for a number of reasons that are pertinent to the ideas I intend to develop in these pages. Before I discuss them, let me state briefly why I now wish to write.

The growing presence in our midst of chemicals that seem to alter consciousness raises questions of the utmost importance for us as individuals and as social beings. Examples of these questions are: What do these drugs tell us about the relationship between mind and body? Are they legitimate tools (in any sense) for changing the mind in a direction of greater awareness? How can a society come to terms with the individual urge to alter awareness? These questions are important because they bear directly on the nature of consciousness, which is, ultimately, the only problem worthy of total intellectual effort. It is the concern of all the world's philosophies and religions, other problems being less precise statements of the same thing. All of us are working on the problem of consciousness on some level, and the conclusions we come to determine what we think about ourselves and the universe, how we live, and how we act. The complex phenomena associated with drugs in our country seem to me to be significant pieces of evidence to be taken into account in this process — clues to help us in our work whether we use drugs or not. It would be useful to have this evidence presented clearly and unemotionally.

In directing attention to matters of consciousness, I am not ignoring or minimizing the very real problems associated with drugs. Our news media are full of documented reports on the tragic consequences of the misuse of chemical agents in search of highs. But having acknowledged the reality of these problems, I propose to find solutions to them by looking to the positive aspects of the drug experience rather than to the negative ones (which are visible all around us). By *positive* I mean simply "tending in the direction of increase or progress" rather than the reverse, and I will attempt to justify this methodology in the course of the book.

During my years as a drug expert (a role I now cheerfully abandon) I have sat through a great many conferences about drugs attended by all sorts of people, but I have never heard the important questions given the attention they deserve. Instead, I have listened to pharmacologists arguing over changes (or possibly no changes) in the chromosomes of rats exposed to LSD, to users rambling on about the purely hedonistic aspects of drug experience, to physicians pretending to themselves that medical science can explain the subjective effects of drugs, to parents and educators begging for methods to make youngsters turn away from drugs, and so on and so on. These discussions have been emotionally charged, but the intellectual level has been uniformly low, whether the participants have been psychiatrists or addicts, students or policemen. I have waited for years for the talk to get around to the interesting questions, but it never has. Nor does it look as if it will. Consequently, I have resolved to stop going to drug conferences and to write instead.

In addition, I have collected an unusual body of information on this subject that I feel obligated to share with people who are interested in the meaningful questions. Through a series of coincidences I have had a chance to look at drugs from the point of view

of a journalist, a user, an ethnobotanist, a physician, a laboratory
pharmacologist, a "drug abuse expert," and a federal government
employee. No one of these viewpoints by itself enabled me to understand what I saw or to come to any useful conclusions. But
gradually, from all the experiences I have had in these diverse positions, certain unifying themes have emerged. And to my great
surprise, the principles that I have begun to discern leave me profoundly optimistic about the possibility of extricating ourselves
from the desperate situation we now find ourselves in. In the following chapters I will describe how I have arrived at certain conclusions and will go into some detail about the reasons for my optimism.

Among the considerations that have kept me from writing until
now, the emotionalism of the subject has been uppermost in my
mind. Drugs are not an emotionally neutral topic of discourse.
There is no such thing as a disinterested drug expert, despite the
stance of many scientists who claim to be presenting purely objective information. This is so precisely because the issues raised by
drugs touch so closely upon our profoundest hopes and fears. Everyone who speaks or writes about drugs (and certainly all who
"investigate" them) together with everyone who hears or reads
what is said and written has an emotional involvement with the
information. The exact nature of this involvement differs from
person to person in both degree and quality, but it is always there.
Consequently, it is extremely difficult to talk about drugs except in
a direct interpersonal situation, where, at least, there is some possibility of monitoring emotional reactions.

In the course of my writings and lectures I have learned that
people hear what they want to hear and tune out what they do not
want to hear.* I have also observed that the distortions of commu-

---

* Here is one example of what I mean. In April 1970 Dr. Norman Zinberg and I published in the British journal *Nature* a paper titled "A Comparison of Marijuana Users
and Non-users," based on interviews with students we had conducted in the Boston
area in 1968. The point of the article was that no personality differences were detect-
able between people who used marijuana recreationally and people who did not in the

nication caused by emotional investments in preconceived notions are most damaging in groups that regard themselves to be
free of such notions, such as physicians and pharmacologists.

Where a topic provokes emotional reactions, one may expect to
see a closely related process of polarization in which divergent interpretations of data develop. The controversies that divide us over
drugs illustrate this process well, for they are not so much battles
over observations as battles over the significance to be attached to
observations. No careful observer doubts that heavy marijuana
smoking correlates with an "amotivational syndrome" character-
ized by lassitude, indifference, and a neurotic inability to accomplish things society considers important. But as soon as we try to
interpret that correlation we run into trouble. Is heavy marijuana
smoking a cause of amotivation, as many psychiatrists tell us, or is
it simply another manifestation of an underlying (and unknown)
psychological process? At every turn in our examination of observations concerned with drugs, we are forced to choose between ri-
val interpretations. What are the real facts?

The answer, very simply, is that there are no facts. Or, more precisely, there are no facts uncontaminated by some degree of value
judgment. Of course, the greater the emotional investments (or
biases) of the participants in this muddle, the greater will be the
degree of contamination. I cannot emphasize too strongly that
everything we hear and read today about drugs is affected in this

---

student communities we studied. We took this finding as an indication of how widespread use of the drug had become — so much so that it cut across all categories; in
other words, students who used marijuana could not be differentiated from other students except by their use of marijuana. By way of comparison we included data on a
group of "chronic users" of drugs — that is, young men who identified themselves as
members of the drug subculture. Here, we did find distinguishing characteristics
(such as a sense of alienation from the dominant culture). In a paragraph of minor importance to the whole paper, we wrote of these chronic users: "There were no signs of
overt intellectual deterioration." As a result of a typographical error, the word *no* was
omitted in the article as it appeared in *Nature*. Despite the fact that the sentence as
printed made no sense, contradicted the rest of the paragraph, and had nothing to do
with the paper as a whole, the *Washington Post* ran a major story the following day under the headline: DAILY POT-SMOKERS ERODE IN INTELLECT, RESEARCHERS CLAIM.

way, all facts put forth about drugs are merely masquerading as such. Nor can I repeat too often that the problem is likely to be most serious in just those cases where it appears to be absent. As I shall show in a later chapter, the pharmacologist who "just gives the facts" about ecstasy, heroin, and marijuana is often interpreting data through the distortions of biases so sweeping and so internally consistent that they remain invisible and unconscious.

These considerations place serious obstacles in the way of anyone who wants to understand what drugs mean. To get by them, we must be carefully discriminating about the information we choose to build theories on. A useful first step is an attempt to estimate the degree and kind of bias present, a practice that should become habitual. To check on the extent of conscious bias, one might ask oneself, Does the person giving me this information have any special case to make for or against drugs? In most instances today the answer will be yes. Law enforcement officers have a personal stake in making drugs look bad; regular users have a personal stake in making them look good. This is garden-variety bias and requires no special aptitude to spot; you just have to remember to ask the question. An affirmative answer does not mean that one should ignore the information, only that one should be alert to the possibility that observations have been interpreted one way rather than another on the basis of relatively meaningless criteria.

Unconscious bias is harder to detect and much more important to try to identify. The question to ask is, Does the person giving this information view the subject from a special perspective that might limit the validity of his or her generalizations? Unconscious bias is as common among proponents of drugs as among opponents. Here are two glaring examples, one from each pole. When I was conducting human experiments with marijuana in Boston in 1968, a Federal Narcotics Bureau agent told me that no matter how my experiments came out, he would remain convinced that "marijuana makes people aggressive and violent." My research had nothing to do with that possibility, but I asked him what his evidence was for his belief. He had one piece of evidence dating from the early 1950s, when he had been seized by a curiosity to watch people smoke the drug. (His official duties were exclusively concerned with large-scale underworld heroin traffic and he had never come into contact with actual users of marijuana.) Accordingly, he had disguised himself as a beatnik and made his way to a Greenwich Village pot party. When he revealed himself as a Narcotics Bureau agent, "everyone there became aggressive and violent." Most people laugh when I tell this story because the logical fallacy is obvious. But when I tried to point it out to this well-meaning man in Boston, he said, "That's what I saw with my own eyes."

In February 1970 I attended a conference in California at which a young, radical sociologist presented data on drug use in American communes. He stated his belief that "marijuana often facilitates the development of communal life." Asked to give evidence on this point, he explained that the question of who was going to wash the dishes was representative of problems encountered in making communes work. He said he had visited communes where this problem had been solved "by having everyone get stoned on marijuana and make a game of dish washing," and he added that "marijuana is known to aid the performance of repetitive tasks." When I objected to this last statement, he replied, "Well, that's what I saw with my own eyes."

Now, suppose we take the trouble to set up formal double-blind experiments on the relationship between being stoned and the ability to tolerate dish washing. We might study two groups of subjects: one would smoke marijuana, the other a placebo, and neither we nor the subjects would know who was smoking what. We would let each group wash dishes. I can predict with confidence that some persons who smoked marijuana would find that dish washing was never so easy. Others would find it harder than ever. Most would find it no different from usual. This pattern of data is very familiar; it comes up again and again in drug research today, and it is one reason why laboratory experimentation on drugs like marijuana has been so unhelpful.

When you ask a question in research and the data come back in this unhelpful way — that is: sometimes yes, sometimes no, most of the time it makes no difference — there is meaning in that result. The meaning is: you have asked the wrong question. In particular, you have tried to make something a causal variable that is not a causal variable. In the case above, the wrongness of the question lies in the hypothesis that the drug has anything causal to do with dishwashing ability. Marijuana smoking and happy dish washing may travel together in some communes, but there is no reason to believe they are more than coincidentally related. It is the attempt to impose a causal relationship on their coincidental association that leads to the framing of a wrongly stated hypothesis. Experiments based on wrongly stated hypotheses uniformly produce useless information.

Most of the research now being conducted on psychoactive drugs is producing useless information at great expense; there is no end of wrongly stated hypotheses. The reason for this state of affairs is logical: precisely because drugs are an emotional subject, drug taking stands out in glowing colors from any complex of behavior of which it is a part. Consequently, observers (even highly trained observers) tend to fall into the trap of trying to explain the entire complex in terms of the drug taking — that is, to make the drug a causal variable when it is not. The tendency to make drugs causes of things we see associated with them is strong in proportion to our emotional involvement, to our unconscious biases. Often it is so strong that it blinds us to obvious factors that are much more directly causative of the phenomena we observe (as in the case of the narcotics agent who was sure that marijuana makes people aggressive and violent). In other cases the attribution of causal roles to drugs is an easy way to cover up ignorance of true causes, which are often more complicated. I suspect, for example, that the ability of some people to wash dishes happily in a commune has to do with a great many factors of personal and social motivation and that the presence or absence of marijuana makes little difference. But we have no ready explanations for variations in motivation from person to person and from setting to setting.

Unconscious biases act like filters between our perceptions and our intellects. They enable us to screen out observations that do not fit in with our preconceived notions and to see causal relationships where none exist. Worst of all, they blind us to their own presence so that we are quick to defend our erroneous hypotheses with shouts of "I saw it with my own eyes!"

I have written at some length about the nature of biases toward drugs in amplification of my contention that it is difficult to communicate accurate information on the subject. Having said all this, I now owe the reader some commentary on my own biases, for, as I have said, there is no such thing as a disinterested drug expert.

I do not have any special case to make for or against the use of drugs. In addition, it will become obvious in the course of the book that my real interest is not drugs at all but consciousness. As for unconscious biases, I am, by definition, unable to identify any I hold at present, but I think I have identified and discarded the commoner ones as I have progressed from one way of looking at drugs to another. For instance, when I was a journalist I thought as a journalist and unconsciously selected from among my observations those that I knew would whet the emotional appetites of my readers. I can give a specific example from an account I wrote for *Look* magazine of the controversy leading to the dismissal of Richard Alpert and Timothy Leary from Harvard University in 1963. In describing the increasing popularity of LSD and mescaline in the Harvard community in the early 1960s, I wrote, "There were stories of students and others using hallucinogens for seductions, both heterosexual and homosexual."[1] Now, there were stories of students and others doing many other less titillating things with hallucinogens, but I picked that one for its journalistic value, and *Look* printed it for the same reason. When I gave up the point

of view of a journalist, I came to see that it was one of the most dis-
torted ways of interpreting observations about drugs, and I resolved not to make use of it again. In my experience the incidence
of serious bias in journalistic accounts of drugs approaches 100
percent; I do not rate scientific journalism any better.

Similarly, I have worked through the unconscious biases of the
pharmacologist and the clinician and have come to see them as
equally limiting viewpoints that prevented me from formulating
useful hypotheses about the effects of drugs. I want to stress the
criterion of "usefulness" in evaluating concepts. The aim of scientific inquiry is not to reveal absolute truth but to discover more
and more useful ways of thinking about phenomena. As philosophers love to remind us, we do not know anything absolutely. For
example, we don't know that the earth travels around the sun; that
is simply the most useful way we now know of interpreting what
we observe — useful because it simplifies things maximally and
thereby gives us greater accuracy of description and prediction
than any other concept yet proposed. If a more useful one came
along, most of us would probably have as much trouble accepting
it as the Ptolemaists had with the heliocentric theory. But more
useful concepts do catch on, however much they are opposed, because they confer a greater degree of success in prediction and
control of the phenomenal world on those who accept them. Their
adherents thus become more fit in the Darwinian sense and have
a distinct survival advantage in the intellectual evolution of the
race.

Our present ways of thinking about drugs are as useless to us as
a geocentric theory of the solar system. They leave us unable to describe, predict, or control the phenomena associated with drugs
except in the crudest ways, as the insoluble drug problem demonstrates. Insoluble problems of this sort are always manifestations
in the physical world of erroneous (that is, useless) conceptual
models. I believe we can literally think our way out of the drug
problem by changing the concepts from which it arises — the out-
moded ways of thinking about consciousness in its ordinary and

nonordinary forms. In essence, then, this book argues that our present ways of thinking about drugs and their effects on the mind have ceased being helpful to us and must be abandoned. I write it as a theorist of consciousness, not as a drug expert, and I will present theories that not only simplify thinking about drug-induced states but also open up possibilities for eliminating the negative phenomena now associated with drugs in our nation.

These theories are original, based entirely on my own observations, and, especially, on my own experience. I cannot see the value of trying to understand consciousness through methods that exclude the most immediately relevant source of information: direct experience of one's own inner states. I am thus firmly on the side of the younger generation in its estimation of direct knowledge above all other kinds of knowledge. Nothing is ever really *known* by indirect means, least of all the nature of one's own mind. My authority for presenting these theories is my own experience, not the medical degree I received from Harvard. In fact, my medical education included not one word on the subjects I shall discuss, and in 1966 my classmates had to petition the chairman of the Harvard Pharmacology Department for a single extracurricular lecture on opiate addiction.

The highly personal nature of some of the experiences from which my ideas have developed has been another source of reluctance to publish this material until it coalesced into a solid theoretical structure. In the following pages I have taken pains to be as frank as possible and to present no hypothesis whose validity I have not checked rigorously against both external and internal observations. My methods place me within a tradition once honored but now disowned by most experimental scientists: that of meticulous self-observation. If the reader will look up a work like Sir Humphry Davy's researches on nitrous oxide ("laughing gas") from 1799, he will find a superb representation of this tradition. Davy uncovered a wealth of useful information about an unknown substance, and he did it with careful intelligence and a spirit of wonder that seems to have vanished from our modern laboratories.[2] Much research today — especially in the areas covered by this book — has become mechanical and dull, more concerned with getting and spending and publishing for the sake of publishing. Real science presses forward on the frontiers of knowledge with a sense of excitement and personal involvement. Like investigators of previous centuries, I have no desire to make my speculations inaccessible to nonscientists. Consciousness is everybody's business because we all carry it about in our heads. I hope that what I am going to say about it will be of as much interest to musicians as to psychopharmacologists; consequently, I have tried to avoid technical language to present these theories in the form of readable chapters built around personal recollections.

For example, in the next chapter I will explore the question of why people take drugs and will introduce the notion of an innate human drive to experience periodic episodes of nonordinary consciousness — a postulate that underlies much of what follows. I have included in this chapter memories of Cambridge, Massachusetts, in 1961, when Alpert and Leary started giving and taking psilocybin. The excitement these experiments generated in the university community and the following that gathered about the two psychologists were clear signs of what was to happen in the nation as a whole within ten years, although few interpreted those signs correctly in 1961. I am not writing history or autobiography. These recollections are merely a starting point for talking about altered states of consciousness — what they are, what their importance may be to us as a species, and what role drugs play in making them available to us. The conclusion I come to in the chapter is that altered states of consciousness have a clear potential for positive psychic development. The drug question can then be restated as a question about methods rather than goals: are drugs the right or wrong means to a desirable end? Accordingly, the chapter that follows is a discussion of arguments that can be made against the choice of drugs as a means to alter consciousness. Certainly, a number of such arguments have already been made. Many of them first came to public attention in 1963 following the

dismissal of Alpert and Leary from Harvard, an event that generated considerable national publicity. But we shall see that most of
the arguments that have been marshaled against drugs have little
basis in logic. It is easy to see why authorities like college administrators get upset at the thought of young people turning on with
chemicals; it is more interesting and much more important to try
to understand why exponents of systems that value alteration of
consciousness (like yoga and Buddhism) take similar positions.

The fourth chapter in this book, "What No One Wants to Know
About Marijuana," is a specific illustration of the ideas developed
in chapter 3. It focuses on the inability of current models of pharmacology and psychology to make sense of the effects of the drug
that is becoming the younger generation's intoxicant of choice. As
a jumping-off point I have used a short account of my attempts in
1967–68 to set up in Boston the first well-controlled human experiments with marijuana.

In the fifth chapter I will take the reader on an excursion to the
Amazon basin for a brief look at societies that use drugs but do
not appear to have problems with them. I offer this cross-cultural
comparison as evidence for my contention that the problems we
have with drugs are not inherent in the drugs but rather in our
ways of thinking about them and about the states of consciousness people seek in them. I believe these South American "primi-
tives" have hit upon basic principles of drug use that are emi-
nently rational and therefore universally applicable, and I will
suggest ways in which they might be translated into terms relevant to our own situation.

"The Solar Mind: Straight Thinking" summarizes conclusions I
have drawn about the nature of ordinary thinking during my years
as a physician and drug specialist, including a year with the National Institute of Mental Health. In these positions I have had a
chance to observe firsthand the shortcomings of a way of thinking
that I believe to be the true source of the problems that seem to be
caused by the use of drugs.

"A Trip to the Moon: Deep Thinking" is a companion chapter

about a very different kind of thinking that all of us have available to us all the time. If we learn to use it, many problems, including the drug problem, will begin to disappear. In this chapter I shall discuss more fully the positive aspects of altered states of consciousness to which I allude in chapter 2, as well as the implications of these theories for other fields of inquiry, particularly medicine and psychiatry.

The eighth chapter is an attempt to use the conceptions developed in earlier chapters and the method of nonordinary thinking to come up with general suggestions as to how we might proceed as a society to come to terms with the drugs that are here to stay.

The final chapter is a brief conclusion that considers the present revolution in consciousness and where it might lead.

I hope this format will allow the reader to trace the evolution of my ideas from the experiences that are their basis. The conclusions I have arrived at did not require any special mental equipment, and I believe their logic will be apparent to anyone who considers the same evidence I have had a chance to go over. I do not regard these ideas as my property in any sense; in fact, I publish them now to make them available to all who care to try them out. Conceptual models are designed for use; after all, that is the only way we will find out how well they work.

I would conclude this introduction with a friendly word of caution. The ideas in this book are revolutionary in the fullest sense of the word. In their underlying optimism and their insistent assignment of a higher priority to consciousness than to the material correlates of consciousness, they diverge 180 degrees from current scientific orthodoxy. Readers who accept my invitation to step through the looking glass may find themselves unwilling to go back, for the paths that open up are many, and they lead to wonders all of us can discover for ourselves.

2. Why People Take Drugs

THE USE OF DRUGS TO ALTER CONSCIOUSNESS is nothing new. It has been a feature of human existence in all places on the earth and in all ages of history. In fact, to my knowledge, the only people lacking a traditional intoxicant are Inuit, who had the misfortune to be unable to grow anything and had to wait for white men to bring them alcohol. Alcohol, of course, has always been the most commonly used drug simply because it does not take much effort to discover that the consumption of fermented juices produces interesting variations from ordinary consciousness.

The ubiquity of drug use is so striking that it must represent a basic human appetite. Yet many Americans seem to feel that the contemporary drug scene is something new, something qualitatively different from what has gone before. This attitude is peculiar because all that is really happening is a change in drug preference. There is no evidence that a greater percentage of Americans are taking drugs, only that some Americans have come to prefer illegal drugs like marijuana and psychedelics to alcohol. Therefore, people who insist that everyone is suddenly taking drugs must not see alcohol in the category of drugs. Evidence that this is precisely the case is abundant, and it provides another example of how emotional biases lead us to formulate unhelpful conceptions. Drug taking is bad. We drink alcohol. Therefore alcohol is not a drug. It is, instead, a "pick me up," a "thirst quencher," a "social lubricant," "an indispensable accompaniment to fine food," and a variety of other euphemisms. Or, if it is a drug, at least it is not one of those bad drugs that other people use.

This attitude is quite prevalent in the adult population of America, and it is an unhelpful formulation for several reasons. In the first place, alcohol is very much a drug by all medical criteria, causing significant alterations of nervous functioning regardless of what euphemistic guise it appears in. In fact, as I will make clear in the next chapter, of all the drugs being used in our society, alcohol has the strongest claim to the label *drug* in view of the prominence of its short- and long-term physical effects. In addition, thinking of alcohol as something other than a drug leads us to frame wrong hypotheses about what is going on in America. We are spending much time, money, and intellectual energy trying to find out why people are taking drugs, but, in fact, what we are doing is trying to find out why some people are taking some drugs that we disapprove of. No useful answers can come out of that sort of inquiry; the question is improperly phrased.

Of course, many theories have been put forward. People are taking drugs to escape, to rebel against parents and other authorities, in response to tensions over foreign wars or domestic crises, in imitation of their peers, and so on and so on. No doubt, these considerations do operate on some levels (for instance, they may shape the forms of illegal drug use by some people), but they are totally inadequate to explain the universality of drug use by human beings. To come up with a valid explanation, we simply must suspend our value judgments about kinds of drugs and admit (however painful it might be) that the glass of beer on a hot afternoon and the bottle of wine with a fine meal are no different in kind from the joint of marijuana or the snort of cocaine; nor is the evening devoted to cocktails essentially different from the evening devoted to ecstasy. All are examples of the same phenomenon: the use of chemical agents to induce alterations in consciousness. What is the meaning of this universal phenomenon?

It is my belief that the desire to alter consciousness periodically is an innate, normal drive analogous to hunger or the sexual drive. Note that I do not say "desire to alter consciousness by means of chemical agents." Drugs are merely one means of satisfying this drive; there are many others, and I will discuss them in due course. In postulating an inborn drive of this sort, I am not advancing a proposition to be proved or disproved but simply a model to be tried out for usefulness in simplifying our understanding of our observations. The model I propose is consistent with observable evidence. In particular, the omnipresence of the phenomenon argues that we are dealing not with something socially or culturally based but rather with a biological characteristic of the species. Furthermore, the need for periods of nonordinary consciousness begins to be expressed at ages far too young for it to have much to do with social conditioning. Anyone who watches very young children without revealing his presence will find them regularly practicing techniques that induce striking changes in mental states. Three- and four-year-olds, for example, commonly whirl themselves into vertiginous stupors. They hyperventilate and have other children squeeze them around the chest until they faint. They also choke each other to produce loss of consciousness.

To my knowledge these practices appear spontaneously among children of all societies, and I suspect they have done so throughout history as well. In our society, children quickly learn to keep this sort of play out of sight of grownups, who instinctively try to stop them. The sight of a child being throttled into unconsciousness scares the parent, but the child seems to have a wonderful time; at least, he goes right off and does it again. Psychologists have paid remarkably little attention to these activities. Some Freudians have noted them and called them "sexual equivalents," suggesting that they are somehow related to the experience of orgasm. But merely labeling a phenomenon does not automatically increase our ability to describe, predict, or influence it; besides, our understanding of sexual experience is too primitive to help us much.

Growing children engage in extensive experimentation with mental states, usually in the direction of loss of waking consciousness. Many of them discover that the transition zone between

waking and sleep offers many possibilities for unusual sensations, such as hallucinations and out-of-the-body experiences, and
they look forward to this period each night. (And yet, falling asleep
becomes suddenly frightening at a later age, possibly when the
ego sense has developed more fully. We will return to this point in
a moment.) It is only a matter of time before children find out that
similar experiences may be obtained chemically; many of them
learn it before the age of five. The most common route to this
knowledge is the discovery that inhalation of the fumes of volatile
solvents in household products induces experiences similar to
those caused by whirling or fainting. An alternate route is introduction to general anesthesia in connection with a childhood operation — an experience that invariably becomes one of the most
vivid early memories.

By the time most American children enter school they have already explored a variety of altered states of consciousness and usually know that chemical substances are one doorway to this fascinating realm. They also know that it is a forbidden realm in that
grownups will always attempt to stop them from going there if
they catch them at it. But, as I have said, the desire to repeat these
experiences is not mere whim; it looks like a real drive arising
from the neurophysiological structure of the human brain. What,
then, happens to it as the child becomes more and more involved
in the process of socialization? In most cases, it goes underground. Children learn very quickly that they must pursue antisocial behavior patterns if they wish to continue to alter consciousness regularly. Hence the secret meetings in cloakrooms, garages,
and playground corners where they can continue to whirl, choke
each other, and, perhaps, sniff cleaning fluids or gasoline.

As the growing child's sense of self is reinforced more and
more by parents, school, and society at large, the drive to alter consciousness may go underground in the individual as well. That is,
its indulgence becomes a very private matter, much like masturba-
tion. Furthermore, in view of the overwhelming social pressure
against such indulgence and the strangeness of the experiences

from the point of view of normal, ego-centered consciousness, many children become quite frightened of episodes of nonordinary awareness and very unwilling to admit their occurrence. The development of this kind of fear may account for the change from looking forward to falling asleep to being afraid of it; in many cases it leads to repression of memories of the experiences.

Yet coexisting with these emotional attitudes is always the underlying need to satisfy an inner drive. In this regard, the Freudian analogy to sexual experience seems highly pertinent. Like the cyclic urge to relieve sexual tension (which probably begins to be felt at much lower ages than many think), the urge to suspend ordinary awareness arises spontaneously from within, builds to a peak, finds relief, and dissipates — all in accordance with its own intrinsic rhythm. The form of the appearance and course of this desire is identical to that of sexual desire. And the pleasure, in both cases, arises from relief of accumulated tension. Both experiences are thus self-validating; their worth is obvious in their own terms, and it is not necessary to justify them by reference to anything else. In other words, episodes of sexual release and episodes of suspension of ordinary consciousness feel good; they satisfy an inner need. Why they should feel good is another sort of question, which I will try to answer toward the end of this chapter. In the meantime, it will be useful to keep in mind the analogy between sexual experience and the experience of altered consciousness (and the possibility that the former is a special case of the latter rather than the reverse).

Despite the accompaniment of fear and guilt, experiences of nonordinary consciousness persist into adolescence and adult life, although awareness of them may diminish. If one takes the trouble to ask people if they have ever had strange experiences at the point of falling asleep, many adults will admit to hallucinations and feelings of being out of their bodies. Significantly, most will do this with a great sense of relief at being able to tell someone else about it and at learning that such experiences do not mark them as psychologically disturbed. One woman who listened to a lecture I gave came up to me afterward and said, "I never knew other people had things like that. You don't know how much better I feel." The fear and guilt that reveal themselves in statements of this sort doubtless develop at early ages and probably are the source of the very social attitudes that engender more fear and guilt in the next generation. The process is curiously circular and self-perpetuating.

There is one more step in the development of adult attitudes toward consciousness alteration. At some point (rather late, I suspect), children learn that social support exists for one method of doing it — namely, the use of alcohol — and that if they are patient, they will be allowed to try it. Until recently, most persons who reached adulthood in our society were content to drink alcohol if they wished to continue to have experiences of this sort by means of chemicals. Now, however, many people have discovered that other chemicals may be preferable. After all, this is what drug users themselves say: that certain illegal substances give better highs than alcohol. This is a serious claim, worthy of serious consideration. We will evaluate it later in this book.

At this point, I would like to summarize the main ideas I have presented so far and then illustrate them with personal examples. We seem to be born with a drive to experience episodes of altered consciousness. This drive expresses itself at very early ages in all children in activities designed to cause loss or major disturbance of ordinary awareness. To an outside, adult observer these practices may seem perverse and even dangerous, but in most cases adults have simply forgotten their own identical experiences as children. As children grow, they explore many ways of inducing similar changes in consciousness and usually discover chemical methods before they enter school. Overwhelming social pressures against public indulgence of this need force children to pursue antisocial, secretive behavior patterns in their explorations of consciousness. In addition, the development of a strong ego sense in this social context often leads to fear and guilt about the desire for periods of altered awareness. Consequently, many youngsters come to indulge this desire in private or to repress it. Finally, older children come to understand that social support is available for chemical satisfaction of this need by means of alcohol. Now, many people, in their continuing experimentation with methods of changing awareness, have come across a variety of other chemicals, which they prefer to alcohol. Thus, use of illegal drugs is nothing more than a logical continuation of a developmental sequence going back to early childhood. It cannot be isolated as a unique phenomenon of adolescence, of contemporary America, of cities, or of any particular social or economic class.

I feel confident about this development scheme for two reasons. First, I have seen it clearly in the histories of many hundreds of drug users I have interviewed and known.* Second, I have experienced it myself. I was an avid whirler and could spend hours collapsed on the ground with the world spinning around — this despite the obvious unpleasant side effects of nausea, dizziness, and sheer exhaustion (the only aspects of the experience visible to grownups). From my point of view these effects were incidental to a state of consciousness that was extraordinarily fascinating — more interesting than any other state except the one I entered at the verge of sleep. I soon found out that my spinning made grownups upset; I learned to do it with other neighborhood children in out-of-the-way locations, and I kept it up until I was nine or ten. At about the age of four, like most members of my generation, I had my tonsils out, and the experience of ether anesthesia (administered by the old-fashioned open-drop method) remains

---

* When I was a student at Harvard many of my friends and associates used drugs and discussed them with me. I began to publish articles on drugs while still in college and became known as a drug expert before I entered medical school, which led other users to seek me out for advice. In 1968 I conducted formal interviews of users in the Boston area in an effort to recruit subjects for laboratory experiments on marijuana. Publicity surrounding publication of these experiments while I was an intern in San Francisco brought numbers of users to me as patients. As a volunteer physician at the Haight-Ashbury Medical Clinic I saw many more users before finishing my clinical training. Since then I have continued to discuss drugs with persons who use them in a variety of settings. It has been my experience that users are delighted to talk about drugs with anyone willing to listen.

one of my strongest memories of early life. It was frightening, intensely interesting, and intimately bound up with my thoughts about death. Some years later I discovered that a particular brand of cleaning fluid in the basement of my house gave me a similar experience, and I sniffed it many times, often in the company of others my age. I could not have explained what I was doing to anyone; the experience was interesting rather than pleasant, and I knew it was important to me to explore its territory.

Alcohol was not forbidden in my home; I was even allowed occasional sips of cocktails or after-dinner cordials. Because I never liked the taste of alcohol, I was unable to understand why grownups drank it so often. I never connected it with my own chemical experiences. I did not discover a real alcohol high until I was a senior in high school; then at age sixteen it suddenly became clear to me what alcohol was — another method, and a powerful one, of entering that interesting realm of consciousness. Soon I fell into a pattern of weekend drinking parties at which everybody consumed alcohol in order to get drunk. These highs were enjoyable for a time, but once their novelty wore off, I indulged in them for purely social reasons. Before long, I began to find the objective, physical effects of alcohol unpleasant and hard to ignore. I hardly knew of the existence of illegal drugs and would not have considered trying them. To me, marijuana was a narcotic used by criminals, and I had no idea why anyone would take amphetamines or opiates.

In the summer of 1960, just before I entered Harvard College as a freshman, I read an article in the Philadelphia *Evening Bulletin* about the death of a student at a southern California college supposedly from an overdose of mescaline. He had been taking it "to get inspiration for papers in a creative writing course." A paragraph from a recent paper was quoted — a visionary description of "galaxies of exploding colors." Mescaline was identified as an experimental drug, largely unknown, said to produce visions. My curiosity was aroused at once, and I resolved to devote my ingenuity to getting and trying mescaline.

At Harvard, excessive weekend consumption of alcohol by students and faculty was the rule rather than the exception, and I went along with the majority even though the experience of being high on alcohol had long since ceased being interesting to me in my explorations of consciousness. Use of illegal drugs was nonexistent except in a very submerged underground. I read everything I could find in scientific journals about mescaline, and then came across Aldous Huxley's famous essay, *Doors of Perception.* The little book convinced me that my intuitions about mescaline as something to be checked out were right. For example, I read:

> . . . [mescaline] changes the quality of consciousness more profoundly and yet is less toxic than any other substance in the pharmacologist's repertory.[1]

And:

> . . . it had always seemed to me possible that, through hypnosis, for example, or autohypnosis, by means of systematic meditation, or else by taking the appropriate drug, I might so change my ordinary mode of consciousness as to be able to know, from the inside, what the visionary, the medium, the mystic were talking about.[2]

Huxley made a convincing case that mescaline was the appropriate drug. Coincidentally, he appeared at the Massachusetts Institute of Technology that fall to give a series of Saturday lectures on visionary experience that were broadcast on the Harvard radio station. I listened carefully to Huxley's thesis that altered states of consciousness included the highest forms of human experience and that chemicals like mescaline were the most direct means of access.

> That humanity at large will ever be able to dispense with Artificial Paradises seems very unlikely. Most men and women lead lives at the worst so painful, at the best so monotonous, poor, and limited that the urge to escape, the longing to transcend themselves if only for a few moments, is and has always been one of the principal appetites of the soul. Art and religion, carnivals and saturnalia, dancing

and listening to oratory — all these have served, in H. G. Wells's phrase, as Doors in the Wall. And for private, for everyday use there have always been chemical intoxicants. All the vegetable sedatives and narcotics, all the euphorics that grow on trees, the hallucinogens that ripen in berries or can be squeezed from roots — all, without exception, have been known and systematically used by human beings from time immemorial. And to these natural modifiers of consciousness, modern science has added its quota of synthetics . . .[3]

As a project for David Riesman's course on American society, I began to write a long study of psychoactive drugs and social attitudes toward them. An instructor in the course suggested that I look up a psychologist, Timothy Leary, who, he thought, was actually doing research with hallucinogens.

I first talked with Leary in his tiny office in the Center for Personality Research on Divinity Avenue. He spoke with sincerity, conviction, and enthusiasm about the potential of drugs like LSD, psilocybin, and mescaline. He envisioned a graduate seminar based on regular consumption of hallucinogens alternating with intensive periods of analysis to identify and apply the insights gained while high. He predicted that within ten years everyone would be using the drugs "from kindergarten children on up." And he did not anticipate strong opposition by society. I asked whether I could be a subject in his psilocybin studies. He said no, he was sorry, but he had promised the university administration not to use undergraduates. He encouraged me to try to get mescaline, which he thought would be possible.

It took two months and only moderate ingenuity to obtain legally a supply of mescaline from an American chemical firm. Then seven other undergraduates and I began taking mescaline and evaluating our experiences with great care. A dozen experiences I had with the drug in 1961 (in half-gram doses) were highly varied. Most were nothing more than intensifications of preexisting moods with prominent periods of euphoria. Only a small percentage of the time did the sensory changes (such as constant motion of boundary lines and surfaces or vivid imagery seen with the

eyes closed) seem worth paying much attention to. In a few instances I experienced great intellectual clarity at the peak of the effect and gained insights that have had lasting importance. After a
dozen trips I was able to see that much of the mescaline experience was not really so wonderful: the prolonged wakefulness, for
example, and the strong stimulation of the sympathetic nervous
system with resultant dilated eyes, cold extremities, and stomach
butterflies. Yet its potential for showing one good ways of interpreting one's own mind seemed enormous. Why was that potential realized so irregularly?

During the year that our drug ring operated out of Claverly Hall,
I had a chance to watch perhaps thirty mescaline experiences of
other undergraduates, and, again, what was most striking was the
variability of these sessions. All of the experiences were mostly
pleasant, with no bad reactions, but no two were alike, even in the
same person. What we were seeing was also being noted by Leary
and Alpert in their continuing studies with psilocybin. They gave
the drug to large numbers of intellectuals, artists, alcoholics, prisoners, addicts, and graduate students; reported that the vast majority of the experiences were positive; and pointed out the importance of "set" and "setting" in determining the subject's reaction.
Set is a person's expectations of what a drug will do to him, considered in the context of his whole personality. Setting is the environment, both physical and social, in which a drug is taken. Leary and
Alpert were the first investigators of psychedelic drugs to insist on
the importance of these two variables. Without them, we are unable to explain simply why there is so much variation in psychic
effects from person to person and from time to time in the same
person. With these variables, the observations become suddenly
clear; hence the usefulness of the concept of set and setting.

I will discuss this concept and its implications when I talk about
marijuana. At this point I will merely note that the combined effects of set and setting can easily overshadow the pharmacological
effects of a drug as stated in a pharmacology text. One can arrange
set and setting so that a dose of an amphetamine will produce se-

dation or a dose of a barbiturate, stimulation. The first time I tried mescaline, my set included so much anxiety (a roomful of people sat around watching to see what would happen) that I felt nothing whatever for four hours after swallowing the dose and thereafter only strong physical effects. There were simply no psychic effects to speak of. This phenomenon has been reported often with marijuana (which I did not try until two years later) and is of great significance, for it argues that the *experience* associated with use of a drug may not be as causally related to the drug as it appears to be.

It is not my purpose here to recount my drug experiences. I write of them to indicate that the route to mescaline, for me and others, was a highly logical one traceable back to earliest childhood. My desire to try mescaline once I had learned of its existence was as natural as my desire to whirl myself into dizziness, hallucinate while falling asleep, sniff cleaning fluid, or get drunk in high school. I did not take mescaline because I went to Harvard, met Timothy Leary, rebelled against my parents, was amotivated, or sought escape from reality. I took it because I was a normal American teenager whose curiosity had survived thirteen years of American education. And it is instructive to note that the way mescaline first came to my attention was through a scare story in a newspaper describing a fatal reaction to the drug (a most improbable event as it turns out).

Now when I say that people take drugs in response to an innate drive to alter consciousness, I do not make any judgment about the taking of drugs. The drive itself must not be equated with the forms of its expression. Clearly, much drug taking in our country is negative in the sense that it is ultimately destructive to the individual and therefore to society. But this obvious fact says nothing about the intrinsic goodness or badness of altered states of consciousness or the need to experience them. Given the negativity of much drug use, it seems to me there are two possibilities to consider: (1) altered states of consciousness are inherently undesirable (in which case, presumably, the drive to experience them

should be thwarted); or (2) altered states of consciousness are neither desirable nor undesirable of themselves but can take bad
forms (in which case the drive to experience them should be chan-
neled in some "proper" direction). Do we have enough evidence to
make an intelligent choice between these possibilities?

Primarily, we need more information about altered states of
consciousness. Altered from what? is a good first question. The
answer is: from ordinary waking consciousness, which is "normal" only in the strict sense of "statistically most frequent"; there
is no connotation of "good," "worthwhile," or "healthy." Sleep and
daydreaming are examples of altered states of consciousness, as
are trance, hypnosis, meditation, general anesthesia, delirium,
psychosis, mystic rapture, and the various chemical "highs." If we
turn to psychology or medicine for an understanding of these
states, we encounter a curious problem. Western scientists who
study the mind tend to study the objective correlates of consciousness rather than consciousness itself. In fact, because consciousness is nonmaterial, there has been great reluctance to accord it
the reality of a laboratory phenomenon; psychologists, therefore,
do not study consciousness directly, only indirectly, as by monitoring the physiological responses or brain waves of a person in a
hypnotic trance or in meditation. Nonmaterial things are considered inaccessible to direct investigation if not altogether unreal.
Consequently, there has been no serious attempt to study altered
states of consciousness as such.*

In the East, psychological science has taken a very different
turn. Subjective states are considered more directly available for
investigation than objective phenomena, which, after all, can only
be perceived through our subjective states. Accordingly, an experiential science of consciousness has developed in Asia, of which
yoga is a good example. It is a science as brilliantly articulated as
Western conceptions of neurophysiology, but no attempt has been

---

* Of course, this has changed since this book first appeared. Academic conferences on
consciousness are now regular events, and new technologies of brain scanning make it
possible to identify neurological correlates of altered states.

made to correlate it carefully with the physical realities of the nervous system as demonstrated by the West.

Therefore, Eastern science should be helpful in understanding altered states of consciousness, but it must always be checked against empirical knowledge of the objective nervous system. Now one of the puzzling and unifying features of altered states of consciousness is their relative absence of physical correlates. For example, there are really no significant physiological differences between a hypnotized person and an unhypnotized person, or even any way of telling them apart if the hypnotized subject is given appropriate suggestions for his behavior. As we shall see, the same holds true for the person high on marijuana — he or she is not readily distinguishable from one who is not high. Consequently, research as we know it in the West really cannot get much of a foothold in this area, and the scientific literature is dreadfully inadequate.

Nevertheless, I think it is possible to come to some useful conclusions about altered states of consciousness from what we can observe in ourselves and others. An immediate suggestion is that these states form some sort of continuum in view of how much they have in common with each other. For example, trance, whether spontaneous or induced by a hypnotist, is simply an extension of the daydreaming state in which awareness is focused and, often, directed inward rather than outward. Except for its voluntary and purposeful character, meditation is not easily distinguished from trance. Masters of meditation in Zen Buddhism warn their students to ignore *makyo*, sensory distortions that frequently resemble the visions of mystics or the hallucinations of schizophrenics. In other words, there is much cross-phenomenology among these states of consciousness, and, interestingly enough, being high on drugs has many of these same features, regardless of what drug induces the high.

The sense of physical lightness and timelessness so often reported by drug users is quite common in trance, meditation, and mystic rapture, for instance. Great ease of access to unconscious memories is also common in these states. Hypnotic subjects capable of sustaining deep trances can be "age regressed" — for example, made to reexperience their tenth birthday party. In deepest trances, awareness of present reality is obliterated, and subjects are amnesic for the experience when they return to normal consciousness. In lighter trances, age-regressed subjects often have a sense of dual reality — the simultaneous experience of reliving the tenth birthday party while also sitting with the hypnotist. Exactly the same experience is reported by users of marijuana, who often find themselves spontaneously reliving unconscious memories as present realities; I have had this sense of dual reality, myself, on a number of occasions when I have been high on marijuana in settings that encouraged introspective reverie.

I want to underline the idea that these states form a continuum beginning in familiar territory. When we watch a movie and become oblivious to everything except the screen, we are in a light trance, in which the scope of our awareness has diminished but the intensity of it has increased. In the Eastern scientific literature, analogies are often drawn between consciousness and light: intensity increases as scope decreases. In simple forms of concentration like movie watching or daydreaming, we do not become aware of the power of focused awareness, but we are doing nothing qualitatively different from persons in states of much more intensely focused consciousness where unusual phenomena are the rule. For example, total anesthesia sufficient for major surgery can occur in deep trance; what appears to happen is that the scope of awareness diminishes so much that the pain arising from the body falls outside it. The conscious experience of this state is that "the pain is there but it's happening to someone else."* I have myself seen a woman have a baby by Caesarean section with no medication; hypnosis alone was used to induce anesthesia, and she remained conscious, alert, in no discomfort throughout the operation.

* Patients given morphine sometimes report the same experience.

I have also seen yogis demonstrate kinds of control of their involuntary nervous systems that my medical education led me to believe were impossible. One that I met could make his heart go into and out of an irregular pattern of beating at will. Such men ascribe their successes in this area solely to powers of concentration developed during regular periods of meditation. There is no need, I think, to point out the tremendous implications of these observations. Because we are unable to modify consciously the operations of a major division of our nervous system (the autonomic system), we are prey to many kinds of illnesses (cardiovascular diseases, for example). The possibility that one can learn to influence directly such "involuntary" functions as heart rate, blood pressure, blood flow to internal organs, endocrine secretions, and perhaps even cellular processes by conscious use of the autonomic nervous system is an exciting frontier of modern medicine. If, by meditation, a person can learn to regulate blood flow to the skin (I have seen a yogi produce a ten-degree-Fahrenheit temperature difference between right and left hands within one minute of getting a signal; the warmer hand was engorged with blood and dark red, the cooler hand was pale), there is no reason why he or she could not also learn to shut off blood flow to a tumor in the body and thus kill it. I will elaborate on these possibilities in chapter 7. Here, I merely wish to note them and emphasize their intimate relationship to altered states of consciousness.

Another chief characteristic of all these states is a major change in the sense of ego, that is, in awareness of oneself as a distinct entity. Thus, when we catch ourselves daydreaming, we wonder where we were for the past few minutes. Now it is most interesting that many systems of mind development and many religions encourage their adherents to learn to "forget" themselves in precisely this sense. For example, in Zen archery (an application of Zen technique that can be used as a spiritual exercise) the meditating archer obliterates the distinction between himself and the bow; hitting the bull's eye with the arrow then becomes no more difficult than reaching out and touching it, and the shot is always a bull's eye. D. T. Suzuki, who brought Zen to the attention of the West, has written of this process: "The archer ceases to be conscious of himself as the one who is engaged in hitting the bull's eye which confronts him."⁴ In fact, the ability to forget oneself as the doer seems to be the essence of mastery of any skill. And since the observing ego is the center of normal waking consciousness, the essence of mastery of any skill is the ability to forsake this kind of consciousness at will.

Furthermore, mystics from all religious traditions testify that this same loss of sense of self is an essential aspect of the highest of human experiences — an assertion the Christian might associate with Jesus' words: "Whoever loses his life for my sake will gain it."⁵ In higher forms of yogic or Buddhist meditation the aim is to focus consciousness on a single object or thought and then to erase all notion of anyone doing the meditation. Patanjali, the ancient writer who first codified and recorded the principles of the much more ancient science of yoga, wrote of *samadhi* (the highest state of consciousness envisioned in yoga): "When alone the object of contemplation remains and one's own form is annihilated, this is known as *samadhi*."⁶ *Samadhi* is a real experience that has been attained by many.

It is noteworthy that most of the world's highest religious and philosophic thought originated in altered states of consciousness in individuals (Gautama, Paul, Mohammed, etc.). It is also noteworthy that creative genius has long been observed to correlate with psychosis and that intuitive genius is often associated with daydreaming, meditation, dreaming, and other nonordinary modes of consciousness.

What conclusions can we draw from all this information? At the least, it would seem, altered states of consciousness have great potential for strongly positive psychic development. They appear to be the ways to more effective and fuller use of the nervous system, to development of creative and intellectual faculties, and to attainment of certain kinds of thought that have been deemed exalted by all who have experienced them.

So there is much logic in our being born with a drive to experiment with other ways of experiencing our perceptions, in particular to get away periodically from ordinary, ego-centered consciousness. It may even be a key factor in the present evolution of the human nervous system. But our immediate concern is the anxiety certain expressions of this drive are provoking in our own land, and we are trying to decide what to make of altered states of consciousness. Clearly, they are potentially valuable to us, not inherently undesirable as in our first hypothesis. They are also not abnormal in that they grade into states all of us have experienced. Therefore, to attempt to thwart this drive would probably be impossible and might be dangerous. True, it exposes the organism to certain risks, but ultimately it can confer psychophysical superiority. To try to thwart its expression in individuals and in society might be psychologically crippling for people and evolutionarily suicidal for the species. I would not want to see us tamper with something so closely related to our curiosity, our creativity, our intuition, and our highest aspirations.

If the drive to alter consciousness is potentially valuable and the states of altered consciousness are potentially valuable, then something must be channeling that drive in wrong directions for it to have negative manifestations in our society. By the way, I do not equate all drug taking with negative manifestations of the drive to alter consciousness. Drug use becomes negative or abusive only when it poses a serious threat to health or to social or psychological functioning. Failure to distinguish drug use from drug abuse — another unhelpful conception arising from emotional bias — has become quite popular, especially in federal government propaganda. The National Institute of Mental Health has labeled every person who smokes marijuana an abuser of the drug, thus creating an insoluble marijuana problem of enormous proportions. Professional legal and medical groups also contribute to this way of thinking. In fact, the American Medical Association has gone so far as to define drug abuse as any use of a "drug of abuse" without professional supervision — an illustration of the peculiar logic necessary to justify conceptions based on emotional rather than rational considerations.

Certainly, much drug use is undesirable, despite the claims of drug enthusiasts, although this problem seems to me much less disturbing than the loss to individuals and to society of the potential benefits of consciousness alteration in positive directions. But let us not get ahead of ourselves. Our inquiry in this chapter is directed to the question of why people take drugs. I have tried to demonstrate that people take drugs to satisfy an inner need for experiencing other modes of consciousness and that whether the drugs are legal or illegal is an unimportant consideration. To answer the question most succinctly: people take drugs because they work.

Or, at least, they seem to.

3. Is Anything Wrong with It?

A GREAT MANY ARGUMENTS are being made against the use of drugs. I hear them on the radio throughout the day and can read them in innumerable pamphlets and books now being showered on young people. But when I pay close attention to these arguments, I find that most of them are directed against consciousness alteration itself rather than against a specific technique. In other words, people fail to distinguish between the method (drug use) and the goal (changing consciousness). This confusion is very common. In my experience it is especially prominent among drug educators, pharmacologists, the administrators of government agencies concerned with drugs, and the drug researchers now supported by government funds. It is an unfortunate confusion because it contaminates the question of the usefulness or harmfulness of drugs with other issues that are highly emotional, as we have seen.

If we are to make any headway in solving the drug problem, we must strictly observe certain rules of evidence. The most important is to identify and remove from consideration all nonessential issues that trigger emotional responses. Once we can see that consciousness alteration is not in itself undesirable, we need be concerned only with an evaluation of methods of achieving it. By carefully distinguishing between method and goal, we will be able to come to conclusions based on reason about the advantages or disadvantages of using drugs. If we fail to make the distinction, the question is wrongly stated, and we find ourselves back on the familiar ground of bias, polarization, and emotion.

A great many arguments against drugs turn out to be inadmissible. For example, the slogan that drugs are an "escape from reality" is really a heavily biased statement about consciousness change in which "reality" is equated with ordinary waking consciousness. It is simply another expression of the fear and guilt all of us have; hence, it is above all emotional and obstructive of the rational process. Another kind of inadmissible argument is one based on circular logic: drugs are illegal because they are bad; therefore, they are bad because they are illegal. Most of the social arguments against drugs are built upon this kind of circularity. The contention that heroin use leads to crime, for instance, is of no help in evaluating the drug because it is impossible to use heroin and not be a criminal in our society. In addition, evidence that drugs are harmful to society has little bearing on the individual decision to use drugs to alter consciousness, and we are interested here in the individual decision.

If we weed out all the inadmissible evidence, we are left with three classes of arguments against drugs: medical, psychological, and practical. The medical arguments have been proposed by doctors and disseminated by law enforcement agents and government administrators; in essence they say drugs can hurt you physically. The psychological arguments (drugs can hurt your mind) come from many sources, notably psychiatrists, and are the mainstay of contemporary drug education. The practical arguments (drugs can hinder you in developing your consciousness) come mainly from former users, exponents of systems like yoga, and religious leaders. I would like to go through these three classes, one by one, analyzing each.

The medical arguments are the easiest to discuss because they diverge from fact so greatly. In general, the illegal drugs that are popular today are not medically dangerous, at least in comparison with legal drugs in widespread use: alcohol, tobacco, coffee, and all the uppers and downers dispensed on medical prescription or sold over the counter in drugstores. No illegal drug is nearly as addictive as tobacco in the form of cigarettes. No illegal drug approaches alcohol in medical harmfulness. These statements will seem startling only if we cling to our biases; they are based on clear observational data.

As a case in point, let us compare alcohol with heroin, which many Americans consider the worst drug one can use — the end stage of a drug progression said to begin with marijuana. Alcohol is representative of a class of drugs known to pharmacologists as "sedative-hypnotics" — a grouping that also includes the barbiturates and the antianxiety drugs that are promoted by pharmaceutical companies and are widely prescribed by doctors.* Heroin is representative of another class of drugs known as narcotics, most of which are derivatives of morphine or other constituents of opium. Both sedative-hypnotics and narcotics are associated with stubborn forms of dependence, often at the expense of health and productivity. But we are interested in determining how much of this association is causal — that is, to what extent the bad effects of alcoholism and heroin addiction are due to the drugs themselves and not to other factors.

Superficially, the two drugs resemble each other. Both are depressants of the activity of the central nervous system (brain and spinal cord). Regular use of both is associated with the two hallmarks of physical dependence: tolerance and withdrawal. Tolerance is the need for larger and larger doses to achieve the same effect. Withdrawal is any syndrome that appears when use is discontinued; by definition it is relieved when the drug is reinstituted.

But here the resemblance between heroin and alcohol ends. Withdrawal from alcohol and barbiturates can be fatal despite medical treatment; withdrawal from heroin is never fatal and is usually unspectacular. I have never seen a withdrawal reaction from heroin that came anywhere near the stereotype promulgated by Hollywood. In fact, I have never seen anyone have as much physical trouble giving up heroin as I have seen many people have giving up cigarettes (which raises questions in my mind about the

* Alprazolam (Xanax) and diazepam (Valium) are familiar examples.

prevailing belief among pharmacologists that nicotine withdrawal is largely imaginary because it has few physiological correlates).* The subjective experience of kicking heroin, like all subjective experiences associated with drugs, seems to be more directly the result of set and setting than of the drug. In a supportive setting, with proper suggestion, a heroin addict can withdraw without medication other than aspirin and have little more discomfort than that of a moderate cold. I saw this in San Francisco in 1968 in men with expensive daily habits.

Tolerance to heroin develops much faster than tolerance to alcohol; consequently, visible dependence on heroin becomes apparent much faster (often in weeks rather than months or years). But the consequences to the body of long-term heroin use are slight compared to those of long-term alcohol use. This is not to say that most heroin addicts are healthy, for most are not. Addicts develop serious acute illnesses — hepatitis, abscesses, AIDS — and often get inadequate medical treatment. In every case, though, the catastrophe has to do with something other than the heroin. The infections come from use of dirty needles and improper injection techniques in people likely to have impaired resistance on account of poor nutrition and irregular lifestyles. On a cellular level, such patients are healthy; therefore, they are satisfying patients to treat medically (if one can ignore their psychological distress) because they can be restored to health with cure of the acute problem — a rare experience in modern internal medicine. By contrast, alcoholics are often sick at the cellular level. They, too, develop serious acute problems (like sudden liver failure and gastrointestinal bleeding), but they cannot be brought anywhere near perfect health no matter how successfully their acute illness is managed. The worst effect on the body of long-term heroin use is chronic constipation. Alcohol induces degenerative changes in liver and nerve function in a significant percentage of its users; our city hospitals are filled with such patients from all social and economic

---

* In fact, recent studies show cigarette smoking to be a harder addiction to break than addiction to either heroin or alcohol.

classes. And the statistical evidence associating alcohol with cirrhosis is at least as impressive as that linking cigarettes with lung cancer.

Many persons die from accidental overdoses of alcohol, usually in combination with other drugs in the same class, like barbiturates. Barbiturates, by themselves, often cause unintended deaths in regular users because tolerance to the lethal dose does not develop as fast as tolerance to the sleep-producing dose. By contrast, accidental overdoses of heroin are the result of irregular cutting and packaging on the black market. If heroin could be isolated from its context in our society, we would soon see that the drug per se is relatively innocuous from the purely medical point of view. Addicts who had access to standard doses of pure heroin, clean equipment, knowledge of how to administer the drug, and good environments would not die of overdoses, develop infections, or contract (and spread) hepatitis and AIDS. Regular use of heroin, even over many years, does not in itself preclude good physical health. Regular, heavy use of alcohol seems to correlate much more tightly with serious medical consequences.

So much for the worst of all drugs. What about the others? For no common category of psychoactive drugs other than the sedative-hypnotics have associations been demonstrated between regular use and direct medical consequences. Many associations have been suggested, ranging from chromosomal damage to brain damage, but all these hypotheses have been based on evidence considered retrospectively. That is, patients with histories of drug use have shown up with various disorders, and clinicians have tried to say that the drug use caused the disorders. Retrospective studies are risky ways of framing hypotheses; they are fraught with logical traps known to the ancients, and it is remarkable that men of science still fall for them.

The saga of LSD and chromosomal damage is a case in point, for much of the evidence was of this retrospective sort. The initial hypothesis, first reported in 1967, was based on the observation that LSD users seemed to have a higher frequency of broken chromosomes in certain white blood cells (lymphocytes) than "normal" persons.[1] The *New England Journal of Medicine* gave this observation great prominence in an editorial titled, "Radiomimetic Effects of LSD," suggesting that the drug mimicked radiation in its damaging effects on genetic material. More circumstantial evidence then appeared: LSD was shown to affect chromosomes of cells growing in test tubes; a few mothers who had used LSD gave birth to deformed babies. The scientific and lay press gave all these findings front-page attention. The National Institute of Mental Health eagerly seized upon and disseminated the new information in a propaganda campaign against LSD. And, for a few months, use of the drug appeared to decline.

But throughout this campaign, a number of facts were overlooked. First was the total absence of any prospective studies supporting the hypothesis. No one had tested the hypothesis in a legitimate way — by looking at chromosomes before exposure to the drug, giving the drug in a controlled fashion, and then keeping watch on chromosomes. Second was the known fact that many things affect chromosomal integrity, among them such common drugs as aspirin and chlorpromazine (Thorazine) and recent viral infections. No effort was made to control for these other factors in the clinical cases. Third was the general problem of tissue-culture studies: cells growing in test tubes do not behave the way cells do in the body. In addition, the doses of LSD that caused visible changes in chromosomes of tissue-culture cells were far higher than the doses living cells get when a person takes an acid trip. Fourth, chromosomal breaks are seen in cells of all people; the arguments turned on a statistical difference in frequency, not an all-or-nothing difference, and the frequency of chromosomal breaks in lymphocytes seems to correlate more directly with laboratory technique than with other variables. (The technique of preparing lymphocytes to make chromosomes visible is complicated and likely to produce factitious changes.) Fifth, the lymphocyte is one of the only cells in which human chromosomes can ever be seen under the microscope. Even if the changes were real, they said nothing about the state of chromosomes in other cells (such as re-productive cells). In fact, through the whole controversy no one showed *why* it was bad to have broken chromosomes in your lym-phocytes. It sounds bad, certainly, but one cannot say that it is bad without making a number of shaky assumptions.

All of these logical flaws in the medical arguments against LSD were obvious in 1967. They do not mean that the hypothesis should never have been published, but surely it should not have been promoted by the medical profession, the press, and the Na-tional Institute of Mental Health without more thought. And it is significant that these logical flaws were first pointed out in the *Berkeley Barb* and other underground newspapers at least eight months before the *New England Journal of Medicine* voiced similar doubts. The necessary prospective studies were not published un-til the end of 1969.[2] Not surprisingly, they failed to demonstrate any relationship between LSD use and chromosomal changes. They generated very little national publicity.

This episode ought to be profoundly embarrassing to journal editors and government scientists. At one stroke it created an ir-reparable credibility gap between users of drugs and drug experts. Since 1968 I have not met a single user of psychedelics who will believe any reports of medical damage associated with these drugs, and the use of psychedelics has never been higher.

A more recent example of the same bad science has to do with ecstasy (MDMA) and neurotoxicity. Dr. George A. Ricuarte, a neu-rologist at Johns Hopkins University and the best-known ecstasy expert in the war on drugs, published numerous animal and hu-man studies claiming to show that MDMA causes brain damage. One, costing $1.3 million and published in 2002 with major pub-licity, stated that the amount of ecstasy consumed in a single night by a typical user might cause permanent brain damage. Over a year after publication, it was revealed that Dr. Ricuarte had ac-tually injected his primate subjects with overdoses of metham-phetamine rather than ecstasy. He explained that labels on two vi-als had somehow been mixed up.[3]

We could go through all the associations that have been suggested between drug use and clinical illness, and in no case would we find a relationship that looks as convincing as that between alcoholism and chronic liver and nerve degeneration. For example, despite decades of argument over the harmfulness of stimulants like cocaine and amphetamines, it remains to be demonstrated that regular use of these drugs causes any physical damage to nerve cells, in the brain or elsewhere. The only exception I would make would be for the volatile solvents (such as those in model-airplane glue) used by some children and adolescents. Heavy use of these toxic compounds may, like alcohol, be associated with liver and nerve problems, but the number of people who actually develop such changes is small. Glue sniffing is an insignificant public health problem compared with abusive drinking.

In fact, the medical harmlessness of most classes of illegal intoxicants — particularly the psychedelics and marijuana — is remarkable. One way of talking about the toxicity of drugs is with a quantity called the therapeutic ratio — that is, the ratio of the dose of a drug that begins to produce toxic symptoms to the dose that produces the effects you want. The therapeutic ratio for most drugs in common clinical use is between 10 and 20. In other words, between 10 and 20 times the dose of aspirin that one takes to relieve a bad headache may begin to cause symptoms of salicylate poisoning. For many drugs in common clinical use, this margin of safety is much smaller. Twice the amount of a digitalis compound given to improve cardiac function can be a lethal overdose. The therapeutic ratio for marijuana cannot be calculated; it seems to be in the order of thousands. On the basis of experiments in cats, one can estimate (roughly) that a possible lethal dose of marijuana for a person of average weight would be a pound and a half taken as a single oral dose. Infants have survived huge accidental ingestions of LSD with no significant aftereffects. LSD and marijuana are among the least toxic drugs known to modern medicine.

The only important medical consequence of long-term mari-

juana use I can see is irritation of the respiratory tract. The problems smokers develop appear to be related more to the amount of
irritation over time than to the nature of the smoke. In general,
even heavy marijuana users inhale far less smoke over time than
moderate cigarette smokers; therefore, they are less likely to develop the lung cancer and emphysema that are so prominently associated with long-term tobacco use. I have heard many people
say: "We didn't know about cigarettes forty years ago; what's going
to happen with marijuana forty years from now?" It is simply not
true that we did not know about cigarettes forty years ago. Many
people knew; no one in a position to do anything listened. Simply
by noting the short-term effects of nicotine (a most powerful drug
with major effects on nerve cells and cardiovascular function) and
the irritant nature of tobacco tars, one could conclude that tobacco
smoking would be a high-risk practice over time. Conversely, it is
our inability to detect clinically significant actions of usual doses
of marijuana that makes me relatively unconcerned about possible long-term medical effects. Drugs that do little to you when you
take them are not going to do more if you take them for a long
time.*

I do not know the effects of marijuana and psychedelics on
pregnancy, but I feel strongly that women should take no drugs
whatever during pregnancy, especially during the first three
months. I also think one can assign relative risk to drugs of concern. I consider LSD a high-risk drug to take during pregnancy,
simply because it is a close relative of the ergot alkaloids, compounds that have significant effects on the uterus. I consider marijuana a low-risk drug to take during pregnancy, simply because it
affects physiological processes so little.

In short, the commonly used illegal drugs — narcotics, psyche-

---

* Concern has been raised about marijuana smoke having a higher tar content than tobacco smoke. Statements like "One joint is equivalent to a pack of cigarettes" are obviously untrue, but certainly there can be harmful effects of marijuana smoking on the
respiratory system. I have seen one case of fatal lung cancer in a sixty-year-old man who
was a regular user of marijuana and never smoked tobacco.

delics, marijuana, amphetamines, and cocaine — are much less dangerous medically than alcohol and less addicting than cigarettes,* both of which we have been living with for some time. I would also rate them much less dangerous medically than many drugs used widely in clinical practice (including some antibiotics and antipsychotics). I do not believe there are any valid medical arguments against the choice of drugs as a means to satisfy the need for periodic episodes of altered consciousness.

The psychological arguments, at first glance, appear to be more convincing. Few attempts have been made to refute them, and all of us have seen psychological casualties that appear to be the results of drug use. For purposes of discussion I will divide these arguments into matters of genuine concern and false issues.

I see two principal matters of genuine concern: (1) the risk of acute psychological disaster; and (2) the problem posed by tolerance.

Any new experience that has the capacity to change one carries a certain risk to psychological stability. The risk of disaster is small but real and it is as true for going to college as for experimenting with sex or entering psychotherapy. In gaining experience, all of us weigh these risks against the potential worth we sense in the new experience. There is no reason why we cannot apply this same way of thinking to drug experience. Is it any riskier than things we are willing to try already?

Three distinct types of psychological disaster can befall a person using drugs. The rarest of these is the toxic psychosis — a nonspecific reaction of the brain to an overdose of anything that affects it. Toxic psychoses are temporary: they disappear when the toxin leaves the body, and they are characteristic of the brain, not of the drug. In other words, it does not matter what drug causes the reaction because the reaction is always the same. The subjective experience of a toxic psychosis is identical to the delirium of high fever,

* Smokable forms of cocaine (crack) and methamphetamine (crystal) are as addictive as cigarettes.

which many of us can recall from childhood. Its characteristic symptoms are confusion, disorientation, and hallucinations, and it is almost always perceived as an unpleasant experience. The condition itself is not dangerous, but it can lead to accidental injury as a result of extreme disorientation. The only treatment is time; as the toxic overdose is metabolized and excreted, the psychological disturbance subsides.

I have, myself, experienced toxic psychoses in response to overdoses of alcohol, *Datura* (jimsonweed), and hashish; the mental effects were the same in all cases. In 1968, when I was studying marijuana in Boston, I deliberately consumed an overdose (6 grams) of potent hashish in order to experience this reaction. I took it orally, under observation, and kept notes as long as I was able. I felt the effects of the drug within forty minutes and found them pleasant but strong for about a half-hour. Thereafter, things became quite confusing. I could not understand what was said to me, felt physically sick, and soon was unfit to do anything but lie in bed and wait for morning. Auditory hallucinations were prominent, especially threatening voices that rose in volume to a crescendo, then faded out. For about twelve hours I remained in a stage of consciousness between sleeping and waking, marked by vivid nightmares. Lucid intervals were rare; for much of the time I did not know where I was, even thinking I was six years old and sick from measles. By morning, most of the worst symptoms had disappeared, but I had a powerful hangover that left me prostrate for another twenty-four hours. I would not willingly repeat the experience.

Any intoxicant can cause a toxic psychosis, but in actuality few do. I have seen them occur in response to amphetamines, psychedelics, hashish (when eaten), belladonna alkaloids, barbiturates, and alcohol. In most cases they result from deliberate ingestion of huge doses, often in an attempt to see how much one can take. In very rare instances, overdoses of drugs may turn up in black-market pills, but, generally, toxic psychoses are richly deserved by those who experience them since they are consequences of reckless use and are easily avoided with minimum intelligence.

The second type of psychological disaster associated with drugs is the panic reaction. It is by far the most common of the three, accounting for nearly all the "bad trips" that come to the attention of psychiatric personnel. Any drug can trigger a panic reaction, but the panic does not seem to have much basis in pharmacology. That is, it is not the direct effect of the drug but, rather, the person's reaction to what he feels the drug is doing to him. First-time users of drugs and persons far removed from the drug subculture are more likely to panic. Also, panic reactions are likeliest in environments where drugs have not yet become established. Many times, only one member of a group panics although all have taken the same dose of the same drug in the same setting. All of these clues point to the set of the individual as the key factor.

The mechanism of a panic reaction is interesting. Initial anxiety (usually conscious) toward the drug makes people interpret their perceptions to mean that they are dying or, more commonly, losing their minds. They then act in such a way as to produce anxiety about their conditions in others and draw upon this anxiety to feed their own. Panic reactions, once they get going, are self-perpetuating and can attain awesome intensity. They continue until the stricken individuals exhaust themselves or until they find someone who does not respond in the usual way. By thinking of panic reactions as drug-induced psychoses, physicians and psychiatrists play into the patient's expectations and often prolong the state. For example, the doctor who administers medication or urges hospital admission for such a reaction unwittingly confirms the patient's fears of a serious condition. I have seen these reactions kept going for up to six days in good hospitals; they can be ended in twenty minutes by anyone who understands their nature.

Persons who have had panic reactions to drugs almost always admit afterward that they could see the panic coming — that is, they were aware of anxiety before they felt the effects of the drug. This is true of panic reactions to anything. In fact, what is important is not that drugs can trigger panic reactions (for anything new can do that) but that people are variously susceptible to panic. Panic-prone individuals can prevent episodes simply by admitting to themselves and others the anxiety they feel in certain situations rather than trying to suppress it. And such individuals should pay great attention to the setting in which they try drugs for the first time. In a supportive environment, panic states do not occur.

Howard Becker, the late sociologist, noted that panic reactions to marijuana, including a few that led to acts of violence, were relatively common as the drug spread into the United States from Mexico after World War I. But from the mid-1930s onward, they began to decline in frequency and eventually became rare. Becker explained the change as an expression of change in expectations (set) toward the drug. When marijuana first appeared in the country it was an unknown quantity. There was no established ritual for its use, no body of folklore to suggest to people what they would experience when they smoked it. Consequently, first-time users in the 1920s probably were much more anxious than their counterparts ten years later, and some of those who expected to lose control did lose control. But as the drug spread across the nation through the nonwhite and Bohemian underground, as it became familiar, individual sets toward it included less anxiety, and panic reactions became correspondingly less frequent. In 1967, when every large city hospital was seeing many bad LSD trips (and most psychiatrists were calling them toxic psychoses), Becker predicted that these, too, would decline in frequency as LSD use increased.[4] And, indeed, this is just what happened, although it was first attributed to the effects of the "new information" about chromosomal damage. Doctors whose only contact with the drug subculture took place in hospital emergency rooms concluded that less LSD was in use when they began to see fewer bad trips. Both the AMA and the National Institute of Mental Health took this position as late as 1970, even though it was clear to most observers of the world at large that use of LSD had never been higher and was still going up. The decline in panic reactions with increasing use of hallucinogens confirmed Becker's hypothesis and emphasized the indirect relationship between the drug itself and the panic reaction associated with it. Because of this indirectness, a person approaching a drug for the first time can take steps to minimize the risk of panic; in fact, the use of common sense in trying drugs reduces this risk to zero.

The third type of psychological disaster associated with drugs in the public mind is the development of a true psychosis. The term *psychosis* is used loosely today, and since it is an emotionally charged word, we had better define it precisely before we begin to discuss it. In conventional psychiatric usage it refers properly to an impairment of a psychological function called "reality testing" — the process by which an individual continually checks his or her interpretation of perceptions against other people's interpretations of their perceptions. If I pass a friend on the street and he does not acknowledge me, I might, in the next few seconds, come up with a number of hypothetical interpretations of his behavior. Some of these might become quite divergent from "reality" as perceived by others, but at some point I would "test" these hypotheses against other sources of information and discard the more unlikely ones. If my reality testing is poor, however, some of these ideas might grow until they become full-blown delusions, just as misinterpretations of sensory data can develop into hallucinations if not checked for accuracy.

It should be clear that no hard-and-fast line divides psychosis from nonpsychosis; all manner of intermediate states turn up. It may be less obvious that psychosis in this sense (that is, the conventional psychiatric sense) may be only one side — the negative side — of an altered state of consciousness, but I think the negativity of the phrase *impaired reality testing* requires no comment. Many thoughtful psychiatrists see that psychosis per se is not a negative alteration of mental function. In fact, the ability to experience reality in unconventional ways may be an unrealized talent in most of us and may explain the empirical correlation between psychosis and genius. I will go into more detail about this possibility in chapter 7. In the meantime I will use the term *negative psychosis* to designate the particular variant of this state of consciousness that is familiar to all institutional psychiatrists. Negative psychotics (for example, schizophrenics) periodically find themselves in trouble with conventional reality, cause confusion in their environments, and usually look upon their own experiences as frightening. They are incurable, according to conventional psychiatrists, hence our natural inclination to want to avoid becoming one.

When a person first comes to be recognized as psychotic, it is often possible to identify a specific triggering incident that precipitated the initial episode of negatively psychotic behavior. For example, the first symptoms of schizophrenia may appear in connection with an emotional upheaval, a change in occupational or marital status, or the start of college. In some cases, clearly, a chemical high acts as the trigger.

But saying that a drug experience can precipitate a psychosis is not the same as saying that drugs cause psychosis. We do not say that sex and college cause psychosis even though we commonly see that both can trigger it. In other words, we acknowledge a potential risk present in sex, college, and many other activities, but we consider the risk a minor aspect of these experiences, especially in comparison with more positive and much more frequent consequences. I see no reason for regarding drug experience any differently. The percentage of users who become negatively psychotic in connection with chemical highs is minuscule — certainly no larger than the percentage of persons who become psychotic in connection with attendance at college. And for most young people today, the potential positive consequences of consciousness alteration outweigh this small but real risk.

Obviously, the decision to use drugs or not will always be a personal decision regardless of social pressures. It should also be an informed decision, made on the basis of all available information.

The risk of negative psychosis is something to be taken into account. But, just as in the case of the panic reaction, this risk is inherent in the individual, not in the external trigger. Psychosis does not come packaged in joints of marijuana, tablets of ecstasy, or lines of cocaine. Rather, people are variously susceptible to developing negative psychosis under stress. What society should do about this possibility — whether it should concentrate on people or on things that can be stressful — is an issue we will discuss when we apply this theory to actual social problems. Here we are concerned with the individual's course of action, and, here again, the risk of this type of psychological disaster does not seem important enough to justify not trying drugs if one is curious about their potential for changing consciousness in interesting directions and knows how to choose a proper setting.

The problem posed by tolerance is the other matter of genuine concern. Anyone who uses a tolerance-producing drug must sooner or later come to terms with the need for larger and larger doses to maintain the experience first associated with the drug. For users of certain drugs this problem comes up much sooner than for users of others, and the problem is very real: the individual must somehow stabilize use in order to keep his or her life from being disrupted by an unstable habit. Unusually rapid tolerance appears in connection with heavy, especially intravenous, use of methamphetamine, even becoming very noticeable within a day or two; its consequences are abundantly clear in urban speed scenes. Disruption of individual lives, social groups, and even whole communities is strongly associated with this particular kind of drug use. For example, the habits of speed freaks are notoriously unstable, taking such forms as "spree shooting" (massive dosing over several days, followed by long periods of exhaustion and semiconsciousness), alternation with periods of heavy barbiturate use, and, eventually, alternation with heroin use. Many observers have noted that large speed scenes (such as the one that developed in the Haight-Ashbury district of San Francisco when the brief era of the flower children came to an end) are inherently unstable and short-lived, always turning into heroin scenes before long. To my mind, this instability is closely correlated with rapid development of tolerance, since methamphetamine taken by injection foils users' attempts to reach equilibrium with their habits. Similar patterns occur when people inhale the vapors of smoked methamphetamine and cocaine.

Equally rapid tolerance to nicotine develops when tobacco smoke is inhaled deeply into the lungs. A high percentage of people who experiment with cigarettes quickly find they cannot stop: they become addicts before they know it. Nicotine is a more powerful stimulant than amphetamine and smoking a more direct way of delivering a drug to the brain than intravenous injection. Most cigarette smokers are able to stabilize their addictions only at high rates of usage, having to put doses of nicotine into their brains every few minutes throughout the day.

By contrast, tolerance to heroin appears more slowly and permits a much greater percentage of users to stabilize their doses. Many addicts never achieve stability with heroin, and they are the ones who come repeatedly to the attention of social authorities, but it is possible that many more persons are hidden addicts who have achieved equilibrium with the drug and thus can lead stable lives (in the same way that many regular drinkers of distilled spirits can stabilize their habits and lead normal lives). Some users, for example, find that they can space injections of heroin far enough apart so that tolerance never gets the better of them. In doing so, they may experience mild withdrawal symptoms at some point during the day, but they are willing to put up with them in order to minimize longer-range discomforts. In other words, stable users, many of whom never are suspected of being users, are psychologically mature individuals; they apply common sense and intelligence to the problem of using heroin. I met some of these people in the San Francisco area in 1969. Most were working-class whites who held steady jobs, bought their drugs with money from their salaries, and led unobtrusive lives in suburbs far removed from what most of us think of as the world of the addict. Some of these people would take one injection of heroin in the morning before going to work and no further doses; others would fix in the morning and evening. Most had kept up these patterns for years.

Tolerance to alcohol becomes a problem over months rather than weeks, but it, too, demands ingenuity and psychological maturity if it is to be contained. In fact, all psychoactive drugs seem to me to pose this problem eventually, including marijuana, and in every case, techniques are available to prevent it from getting out of hand. Whether a user will discover the techniques is, again, a matter of personality — of set and setting — rather than a matter of pharmacology.

Despite massive research efforts, no satisfactory biochemical or physiological theory of tolerance has been proposed. My own guess is that this problem, too, is wrongly stated. Tolerance is not a phenomenon associated only with drugs. In fact, it looks as if human beings become tolerant to any pleasurable experience indulged in too frequently. Therefore tolerance might be an intrinsic part of human experience rather than a purely material change. Its correlates in the material world might well be physical changes in the body and brain, but its causes probably lie elsewhere. I will return to this point when I discuss the practical arguments against the use of drugs to alter consciousness.

To sum up, regular use of any drug is associated with the development of tolerance to the experience. This fact poses a problem because drug use tends to disrupt one's life to the extent that it is unstable. All drugs confront the user with this problem eventually, some in a very short time. One can learn to deal with tolerance and come to equilibrium with the use of any drug, but to do so requires intelligent discovery and application of certain principles of safe interaction with drugs. (I will expound these principles in examining attitudes of South American Indians toward drugs.) The problem posed by tolerance is a legitimate caveat worth pointing out to people starting to use drugs, but it still does not qualify as a good reason for not using drugs to alter consciousness. It is something to know about and to be careful of, nothing more.

And I do not see any other legitimate matters of psychological concern.* All of the other psychological arguments against drugs seem to me to be false issues that have no basis in fact. It is not my purpose to dissect every argument of this sort; instead, I will give examples of the three varieties of false issue and let the reader who wishes extend the list.

The first variety will be familiar from earlier pages. It is the incorrect attribution of causal relationships to correlations between drug use and behavior. One example is the assertion that heavy marijuana use causes amotivation, which I have already mentioned in the first chapter.† Another example is any theory of "drug progression" that states, drug A leads to drug B. It makes no sense that any drug has qualities that lead its users to want to try other drugs.‡ It makes much sense that people who tend to use

---

* A possible concern I should mention is the question of whether there is a critical age below which the use of drugs to achieve highs might be harmful. In the drug subculture it is not unusual for very young children to smoke marijuana or even try psychedelics, but we have no real information on the effects of such use. In primitive cultures future shamans may start exploring drug-induced trances before the age of five, apparently without long-range adverse consequences. In our culture it is possible that too much alteration of consciousness before the ego-sense is well developed might prevent a person from using altered states of consciousness to benefit in later life.

† When I was a freshman at Harvard, long before many people thought of smoking marijuana, there was plenty of amotivation. It took such forms as sleeping till dinner time and then playing cards all night instead of working and was indistinguishable from amotivation now associated with heavy marijuana use. Heavy marijuana use is a convenient symptom for an amotivated person to add to his list: it is fun, can be done with other people, angers grownups, and so on. It is too late to find a rural college where marijuana is still unknown. If one existed, I would predict that the amotivated people there would become the heavy marijuana smokers once the drug appeared on campus. If marijuana were the cause of amotivation, one would expect that amotivation could be cured by taking away the marijuana, but this is not the case. Therefore, it makes more sense to see amotivation as a cause of heavy marijuana smoking rather than the reverse.

‡ Except for stimulants like amphetamines and cocaine, which may encourage users to take sedatives to "come down" at the end of a period of stimulation.

drugs excessively (unstable users) will also be unstable about the kinds of drugs they use. In my experience with patients having drug problems I have repeatedly seen that people who tend to use drugs heavily tend also to use many different drugs, often preferring more potent forms. But I have found it unhelpful to try to read meaning into the sequence by which they go from one drug to another. It is an unhelpful way of thinking because it prevents the formulation of useful hypotheses. The classic ghetto heroin addict smoked marijuana before he tried heroin. But he also did many other things that marked him off as a unique type. Typically, he began smoking cigarettes before the age of ten, was drinking heavily before he tried marijuana. What hypothesis about drugs can we draw from these observations that will have any value?

We saw college students smoking marijuana in large numbers. Then we saw some of them trying heroin occasionally. Did marijuana lead to heroin use, after all? This is *post hoc ergo propter hoc* reasoning, and it does not work whether or not the fallacy is clothed in up-to-date observations. And this famous logical trap is at the heart of most of the hypotheses launched against drugs by negatively biased psychologists. An extraordinary example is the clinical entity called a "flashback," said to be a spontaneous, involuntary recurrence of psychedelic drug effects some time after the drug has worn off. Flashbacks can happen days, weeks, or months after the high, last for seconds or minutes, and frequently provoke anxiety in young patients. They captivated the attention of clinical psychologists and psychiatrists and became the subject of hundreds of scientific papers. Theories were proposed for biochemical and neurophysiological mechanisms underlying flashbacks. Debate raged as to whether they should be taken as a sign of psychological dysfunction.

Throughout this development, some simple observations went unnoticed. Flashbacks seem to be as common among people who have never used drugs as among people who have taken psychedelics. And at least as many people welcome them as become anxious about them. I have asked many non-drug-using young people how often they experience spontaneous, transitory episodes of depersonalization (a sense of losing contact with external reality), derealization (things becoming unreal and weird), and hallucinations. The percentage who admit to such episodes approaches 100. Flashbacks are especially common in school, at work, and between sleeping and waking. They seem to be a normal neuropsychological event, much like the episodic experience of *déjà vu* that everyone knows. Since there is a rough correspondence between the experience of a flashback and the experience of a mushroom trip, it is logical that a user would associate the two at the time of the first flashback following the trip. If he or she were still anxious about the trip, the anxiety would become attached to the flashback by conditioning. Thus fallacious logic leads to the creation of real symptoms, which can be reinforced in treatment by a psychologist who makes the same error. The doctor who comprehends that flashbacks are not causally related to psychedelic mushrooms can take a much more useful approach: he can reassure the patient that the phenomenon is normal and has nothing to do with the trip. The patient's anxiety then diminishes, his attention is no longer focused on his flashbacks, and he is "cured." The success of this method is an example of the real power over phenomena conferred by more useful ways of thinking.

A second variety of false issue is one concocted out of nothing by verbal magic. In 1967, Jerome Lettvin, a well-known psychiatrist, neurophysiologist, and drug expert, argued in an article in *Natural History*[5] (reprinted and distributed by the National Institute of Mental Health) that psychedelics might impair judgment and perception "for a long time" and that "this disorder may be such that the man cannot judge he is disordered." But what are the objective signs of this disorder? Lettvin wrote: "Thus it is that students, already somewhat pressed, already subject to the far less than idealistic tenor of our schools and the nature of our society, on taking such compounds can become easily recruited to the hip-

pies, and turning on, drop out." This statement is heavily laden
with negative value judgments about alternate lifestyles; if we remove them, we are left with the argument: Psychedelics can hurt
your mind including your ability to know that your mind has been
hurt — a line of reasoning that is unhelpful because of its gratu-
itous negativity. The only meaning in it and statements like it is
the real anxiety created in the minds of young people experimenting with psychedelic drugs. In 1969 I saw in the psychiatric emergency room of Mount Zion Hospital in San Francisco a fifteen-
year-old boy who had paralyzing anxiety associated with a three-
week-long depression. He had been going through a phase of using LSD frequently with a friend. Three weeks before, the friend
had been caught by his parents and forced to go to the family doctor for "treatment." The physician told his patient that his use of
LSD had "probably killed off twenty thousand brain cells." Since
then, both boys had been depressed. I asked this patient if he
thought he had lost all those brain cells. He said yes. I asked him
whether his brain felt any different to him. He said no. Then what
real difference did it make? His mind was intact; his only problem
was acute anxiety, depression, and low self-esteem. As soon as he
was able to reassure himself about his mind, his anxiety subsided.
Within a day his depression lifted and he resumed his normal
level of activity. Later, he indicated his intention to try LSD again. I
did not attempt to discourage him but urged him to regard his frequent use of LSD as a phase that he would have to progress beyond in order to continue to extend his experience. He was very re-
sponsive to this approach.

This case shows how ways of thinking that spread anxiety and
pessimism tend to be counterproductive. Good motives must be
linked to right methods.

The third variety of false issue (and perhaps the most interesting) is the negative description — that is, an accurate description of drug-associated behavior but one consistently interpreted
through a negative bias. The concept of psychological dependence
is a product of this kind of thinking because it is simply a negative

way of describing the behavior of someone who does something repeatedly because he likes it. Throughout medical school I was psychologically dependent on Coca-Cola. Many men I know are psychologically dependent on their wives.

Contemporary drug education includes a great deal of this kind of bias. Here is a statement from a recent curriculum for high school students that purports to "give unbiased facts so that students can decide for themselves whether or not they will try marijuana":

> Some people when they smoke a joint and eat a cheeseburger think the cheeseburger tastes better. Actually, this is not so. What has happened is that the marijuana has interfered with immediate memory so that they do not remember what the last cheeseburger they ate tasted like.

Especially disturbing in this example is the underlying assumption that a hypothesized negative effect in the material world is more "real" than an experience in the nonmaterial realm of consciousness. It is an element of the same materialistic philosophy that ultimately denies the reality of consciousness itself.

Negative descriptions of drug users are very common in contemporary psychiatric literature. Consider these examples from an article titled "Chronic Psychosis Associated with Long-Term Psychotomimetic Drug Abuse" written by two psychiatrists at the Connecticut Mental Health Center and published in the August 1970 issue of the *Archives of General Psychiatry*. Drs. Glass and Bowers present cases of young men who have had extensive experience with marijuana and LSD and who have been hospitalized against their wills, typically because their behavior and changing lifestyles began to scare their parents. In presenting the objective signs of their "psychosis" Glass and Bowers include these sentences (about four separate patients): "On admission he had shoulder-length hair, a saddened aged face, and appeared underweight." "He avoided meaningful interaction in a stereotyped manner." "He would sit passively." "His affect was flat and bland."* "Word associations were not loose but revolved around a philosophical belief in Eastern religions, LSD experience, and himself as the passive agent for whom things were cosmically determined." "He was placed on large doses of chlorpromazine† (900 milligrams a day) which had some calming effect but did not alter his basic manner of thinking." "The passive style, preoccupation with Eastern religious fatalism, and avoidance of social interaction persisted." "On a visit home, his parents noted that he was acting and dressing in a bizarre fashion and insisted on his hospitalization." "On admission he was dressed in Chinese robes, wore shoulder-length hair and a beard, and appeared grossly underweight." "His affect was shallow and flat, associations circumstantial and vague, while thinking centered around a desire to love and fuse with others which he phrased in mystical terms." "His thought content centered on an interest in Eastern religions in which one could meditate to reach Nirvana where 'all things are one.'" "We have been impressed with the effect heavy long-term drug use (the periodic production of a uniquely altered state of consciousness) may have upon the resolution of crucial maturational conflicts and the production of a less internally conflicted chronic psychotic state." "All these individuals were withdrawn and isolated on the ward." "Their affect was shallow and thought

* *Flat affect*, a favorite psychiatric term for loss of normal moment-to-moment mood swings, is supposed to be a hallmark of schizophrenia but equally well describes the placidity attained by a student of meditation.

† The phenothiazine tranquilizers, which have "revolutionized" modern psychiatry, have been sold by the pharmaceutical industry and bought by the psychiatric profession as "antipsychotic agents." They are not anything of the sort. Rather, they are special kinds of sedatives that specifically make it hard to think. In practice, they prevent negative psychotics from expressing the forms of their altered state of consciousness in ways disturbing to the staffs of mental hospitals. It is an interesting consideration that of all the drugs used to alter consciousness, antipsychotics are almost never taken except on orders from medical professionals. The experience provided by these drugs is universally perceived to be the wrong direction in which to alter one's consciousness. They suppress the symptoms of negative psychosis much as alcohol suppresses the symptoms of anxiety, and they lead to the same sort of dependence because they do not touch the source of the problem.

processes, while not loose, were bizarre and centered on Eastern religious mysticism." "Electric convulsive treatments were used in one patient with no noticeable effect." "Briefly stated, these patients appeared unfortunately comfortable with their psychoses."

The negative value judgments that occur continually throughout this writing do not require amplification. In my experience with patients having problems with drugs, I have consistently found that if one dwells on the negative side of the patient's personality, one is unable to change his behavior except for the worse. But if one looks for the positive side (which is always there), contact is established, and one can then motivate the patient to use his developing consciousness to solve his problems with the world.

We have seen that, aside from a few matters of real concern, all of which can be handled by the use of common sense, the psychological arguments against drugs turn out not to be real issues. I do not believe there are any valid psychological arguments against the choice of drugs as a means to satisfy the need for periodic episodes of altered consciousness.

But when we turn to the practical arguments, I think, at last, we do find validity. To be sure, many of the pronouncements of religious leaders about drugs are just as biased as those of physicians and psychologists. The assertion that spiritual experiences triggered by psychedelics are "not genuine" belongs in this category. The National Institute of Mental Health has said this; so has Meher Baba, a Hindu sage who died leaving a large following in the West. In a pamphlet titled "God in a Pill?" Meher Baba wrote: "All so-called spiritual experiences generated by taking 'mind-changing' drugs such as LSD, mescaline, and psilocybin are superficial." It would seem obvious that the only meaningful criterion for the genuineness of any spiritual experience — whether or not it occurs in association with a drug — is the effect it has on a person's life. I would be suspicious of a person who had "spiritual experiences" with mushrooms every weekend and kept up all of his old behavior patterns. I would be impressed with a person who manifested spirituality in his life after a profound mushroom experience.

Now it is interesting that people who begin to move in a spiritual direction in connection with drug experimentation sooner or later look for other methods of maintaining their experiences. One sees many long-time drug users give up drugs for meditation,* for example, but one does not see any long-time meditators give up meditation to become druggies. This observation supports the contention that the highs obtainable by means of meditation are better than the highs obtainable through drugs — a contention phrased not in moral terms but simply in practical ones.

It is also interesting that every major religion and system of mind development that stresses the value of direct experience urges the avoidance of chemical highs. Yoga and Buddhism are both very clear on this point, for example, even though both recognize that drugs are effective means of altering consciousness. In his ancient aphorisms on yoga, Patanjali wrote: "The psychic powers may be obtained either by birth [that is, as a result of actions in past lives], or by means of drugs, or by the power of words [repetition of sacred syllables or phrases], or by the practice of austerities, or by concentration."[6] Yet all yoga texts demand abstinence from drugs. The ancient Hindus certainly had available to them alcohol and marijuana; they also had *soma*, the "divine intoxicant" of the Vedas, almost certainly a psychedelic potion made from a plant.

Because yoga and Buddhism developed in cultures so familiar with psychoactive drugs, their followers ought to be able to speak with some authority. In addition, the levels of consciousness sought and achieved by yogis and Buddhists seem to me more impressive than those attained by men who have exhorted their disciples to use drugs. Aleister Crowley, the twentieth-century British occultist, founded a secret order that emphasized drug use; his

---

* Richard Alpert is an example. In his role as Baba Ram Dass, a disciple of a Hindu guru, he has encouraged followers to turn on with yogic meditation rather than drugs.

own life was considerably less inspiring than the lives of many of his contemporaries who pursued the same ends through the standard techniques of Eastern systems. Unfortunately, most spokesmen for yoga and Buddhism state their position on drugs dogmatically. For example, Edwin Arnold in his famous poem, "The Light of Asia," which introduced generations of Westerners to Buddhist thought, gave the fourth of Gautama's Five Rules in this couplet: "Shun drugs and drinks which work the wit abuse;/ Clear minds, clean bodies need no *soma* juice." This typically dogmatic style had made it very easy for users in this country to reject Eastern attitudes about drugs as more establishment propaganda.

Careful study of Eastern literature, however, shows that yogis and Buddhists are strictly concerned with practicalities. Continued alteration of consciousness by means of drugs, they say, ultimately makes it harder for individuals to attain and maintain the most worthwhile states of consciousness. Their reasoning is clear: drug experience strongly reinforces the illusion that highs come from external, material things rather than from one's own nervous system, and it is precisely this illusion that one strives to overcome by means of meditation. Long before I understood this point of view, I had made an interesting clinical observation. I noticed that all persons I met who were visibly dependent on drugs, whose lives were ruled by their habits, thought about drugs in a particular way. They were convinced that the experiences they enjoyed came in the joints of marijuana, tablets of ecstasy, or lines of cocaine, and they saw no other way of getting them. There is no doubt in my mind that drug dependence is essentially an error of thinking, not a pharmacological or biochemical phenomenon, even though it may be accompanied by changes in the physical body. And it makes no difference whether the drug is marijuana, heroin, or alcohol; the error in the mind is always the same.

I am further struck by a curious symmetry between people who abuse drugs and people who study them. The person who is convinced that highs come in drugs, if negatively oriented toward society, becomes a drug abuser; if positively oriented toward society, may become a drug researcher. But the two are essentially the same, because both are laboring under the identical materialistic illusion. Only their mutual antagonism keeps them from realizing they are two poles of the same way of thinking.

People who think that experiences come in drugs eventually find that drugs begin not to work as well for them. This subjective tolerance to experience seems clearly related to an illusory way of thinking, because people who see through the illusion solve the problem of tolerance whereas people who do not are overcome by it. People who begin to notice that ecstasy no longer puts them in the right place as well as it used to have a choice. They can begin to look for other methods of getting to that place or they can pursue the experience through the drug more and more desperately. In the former case, they will evolve away from drugs in their continuing explorations of altered states of consciousness. In the latter case, they will become involved with drugs in a more and more neurotic manner and eventually will become less free to use their nervous systems in interesting ways.

These considerations explain why drugless highs are often perceived as better than drug highs. Drug experience includes many extraneous phenomena that are irrelevant to the desired state of consciousness. For example, when one takes mushrooms and perceives cosmic unity and bliss, it is not essential to have dilated eyes, cold hands, butterflies in your stomach, and prolonged wakefulness. These pharmacological actions of the drug on the lower parts of the physical nervous system are direct effects of the drug; the experience is an indirect effect coming from the mind in response to this physiological trigger. It never occurs to many drug takers that the two aspects of drug experience are separable and that the high can be had without its physiological trappings. But the first time one achieves such separation, the superiority of a pure high uncontaminated by physiological "noise" is obvious. The trouble is that drugs seem to work powerfully and immediately, whereas meditation requires persistence and effort. But the results may be worth it.

Here also is an explanation of the ineffectiveness of methadone as a treatment for heroin addiction. Methadone is a narcotic that produces all the physiological noise of narcotics but that, in clinical settings, does not provide a high. Now, every heroin addict gets a high from heroin, and, however much heroin may disrupt his or her life, the high compensates for the discomfort. In switching addicts to methadone, doctors are asking them to give up this experience for nothing in return — an unreasonable expectation. A more useful approach, it seems to me, would be to show addicts how they can get highs in other ways, even if this means weaning them from one drug to another rather than asking them to abstain from drugs entirely. Oral opium is one possibility. Another is nitrous oxide (laughing gas), which might be helpful because it provides a rush (that is, the experience of going suddenly from one state of consciousness to another) that heroin users seem to like. Furthermore, it is possible to encourage people who have experimented with nitrous oxide to experiment with meditation, whereas the transition from heroin to meditation in one step is very difficult to effect.

The idea that drugs do not really work at all but only appear to has very far-reaching implications for our understanding of the relationship between inner, subjective reality and outer, objective reality. I will comment on some of them later. Right now I will illustrate the principle that drugs only appear to work in a detailed look at marijuana, which, of all the drugs that trigger highs, does least in the material realm. It offers, therefore, the best possible opportunity to see through the illusion that has enchanted both abusers and researchers.

To conclude this chapter, let me summarize my own beliefs: Drugs do not hurt the body in the ways most physicians think; they do not hurt the mind in the ways most psychiatrists think; but they can keep people from reaching the goal of consciousness developed to its highest potential. The subtlety of this risk is worth noting: at the very time that drugs are triggering valuable states of consciousness they are reinforcing the illusion that these states of consciousness arise from external reality rather than internal reality. Thus it is ironic that persons who have the most positive experiences with drugs may also be the ones who become most enmeshed in illusory ways of thinking about their own minds.

4. What No One Wants to Know About Marijuana

I PROGRESSED TO MARIJUANA FROM NUTMEG.
In the summer after my first year of college, I was invited to a "mace party" in suburban Philadelphia given by several of my high school friends who were now attending Haverford and Swarthmore colleges. Word had reached Haverford the previous spring by way of a visiting beatnik that one could get high on mace (the spice obtained from the outer covering of nutmeg seeds); the story was to take one or two tablespoonfuls mixed with fruit juice. We did. We then waited three or four hours but nothing happened, and I went home to bed. Next morning I had a powerful hangover, aching joints, and weak muscles that lasted most of the day.

It seemed incredible to me that a common spice could have such toxic effects; I decided to check up on it when I got back to school. That fall I began an association with the Harvard Botanical Museum and its director, Dr. Richard Evans Schultes, that was to continue for many years. The godfather of modern ethnobotany, Schultes was mainly interested in psychoactive plants, especially those of the New World tropics, where he had made extensive collections. Under his guidance I began an investigation of the pharmacology and ethnopharmacology of nutmeg that led to a term paper, a thesis, and a number of articles in scientific journals. I discovered that nutmeg, mace, and many other spices contain compounds that affect the central nervous system. In fact, the active principle of nutmeg seemed to be a chemical (myristicin) that was structurally similar to amphetamine and mescaline. Nutmeg had a long history of use as a medicinal agent, and, throughout the centuries, cases of intoxication had been noted. At the time of my studies (1962–64) it was used mainly by drug takers who found themselves cut off from supplies of drugs — such as men in prisons. American nutmeg eaters compared the effects of the spice most frequently to those of marijuana.

I first smoked marijuana in 1963; like many first-time users I experienced nothing whatever from it. But a marijuana subculture was definitely in existence at Harvard at that time, and newspaper editors in Boston were discovering that the "marijuana problem" in Cambridge made good copy. The Botanical Museum library had an excellent collection of books and articles on psychoactive plants, including one of the only copies in the United States of the original Indian Hemp Drugs Commission Report, published by the British Government of India in 1894. When I got tired of poring over old herbals in search of information about nutmeg, I would delve into the voluminous scientific literature on marijuana. I could not believe what I found. Although thousands of articles were available on hemp (including hundreds written in English over the past century), almost none of this material had anything to say. It was a vast collection of rumor, anecdote, and secondhand accounts. For example, an American physician who had traveled to India in 1910 and talked with several Indian physicians would publish a paper recounting their opinions about the effects of hemp drugs. Many writers had strong opinions about the drugs, but whenever I tried to trace these opinions back to any sort of basis in experimental observation, there was none to be found. I could discover only three instances in American history when marijuana had actually been given to human beings by doctors to see what it did. The first of these was the Canal Zone study of 1933, prompted by growing popularity of marijuana smoking among American soldiers. The second, in 1944, was the famous LaGuardia study that drew bitter attacks by the Federal Bureau of Narcotics and the American Medical Association. The third, in

1946, was a series of experiments conducted at the Public Health Service Hospital in Lexington, Kentucky. And that was it. No experimental work had been done since 1946. Furthermore, none of the studies on record was satisfactory by present standards of drug testing.

I have already discussed the importance of set and setting in determining individual responses to all drugs. It is possible to arrange drugs on a continuum along which the influence of set and setting becomes steadily greater relative to the influence of direct pharmacological action. At one end would be certain clinical drugs like atropine (given preoperatively to surgical patients to dry up secretions in the respiratory tract), which we have come to think of as having no psychic effects. (What we really mean is no psychic effects we pay attention to or care about.) At the other end are the psychoactive drugs, in which category the psychic component of the individual's response is the focus of attention. Even within this broad category there are gradations. Because they produce noticeable depressant effects on the brain, alcohol and barbiturates strongly influence psychic response by virtue of their direct pharmacological action. Set and setting are important in shaping individual responses to alcohol, but they are much more important in shaping individual responses to marijuana, which, in usual doses, has no clinically significant actions on lower brain centers. In fact, marijuana lies at the other extreme of the continuum — where the influence of set and setting dwarfs the influence of the drug itself.

If you wish to find out what the drug itself does, how can you control for the other factors? The problem is not simple. The setting of a pharmacology laboratory is very special compared to the settings in which drugs are used recreationally. The biases of the experimenters may seriously contaminate the set of experimental subjects, even if no direct verbal communication takes place. One solution is to administer drugs and placebos to volunteer subjects in double-blind fashion: that is, neither the subject nor the experimenters know who has received a drug and who a placebo until the experimenters are finished. (In practice, this can be done by entrusting the information to a third party who prepares identical-looking doses according to a code unknown to the experimenters.) The double-blind method is the only method that protects the experiment from experimenter bias.* Single-blind testing (where the subject is in the dark but the experimenter knows what the subject is given) is not sufficient. But the double-blind method was not generally accepted in pharmacology until after World War II. Therefore, none of the early marijuana studies had made use of it.

It seemed to me, back in 1963, that a simple double-blind human study of marijuana was urgently needed; I resolved to set one up as soon as I was in a position to do so. Not until my last year of medical school was that possible, and even then it was possible only in the face of overwhelming odds. I had six months of elective period at the very end of my medical studies — the only elective time in a four-year curriculum. In the spring of 1967, I notified Harvard that I wished to devote this entire block of time to a research project on marijuana. I also approached Dr. Norman Zinberg, a Harvard psychoanalyst and friend, with the idea; he agreed to be my faculty sponsor. We had a full year in which to get things organized, but that turned out to be barely enough time.

I was under no illusions about the difficulties that had to be surmounted. The legal status of marijuana was, to say the least, confused, with a number of different federal, state, and local agencies claiming jurisdiction. The prospects for coordinating favorable responses from all these bureaucracies were dim. No one in the Pharmacology Department of Harvard Medical School was particularly knowledgeable about marijuana (or about the other drugs that were increasingly evident in Cambridge and Boston), and, besides, Harvard had become quite paranoid about human drug ex-

---

* However, I doubt very much that the double-blind method is *adequate* protection. Nonverbal communication is most powerful and may transmit to the subject the expectations of the experimenter even in the most carefully designed double-blind procedure.

periments in the wake of the Alpert-Leary furor. I was a medical student, not a licensed physician, which further complicated the legality of experiments I would conduct. Several pharmacologists told me outright that no one could get permission from the Federal Bureau of Narcotics to administer marijuana to human beings. A Boston attorney who was pressing a case to test the marijuana laws bet me that I would never succeed.

But Zinberg and I were determined to try. We made contact with a group of pharmacologists and psychiatrists at Boston University School of Medicine who were willing to sponsor the project. They knew something about psychoactive drugs from the viewpoint of pharmacology, and I was hopeful that Boston University would be less obstructive than Harvard. In late summer I approached the Federal Bureau of Narcotics in Washington; the agency's chief legal counsel indicated his willingness to help. Then I spoke with representatives of the National Institute of Mental Health, which had just been given a large sum of money by Congress to get research started on marijuana. To my surprise and dismay, the people at NIMH responsible for this task knew less about the problems of getting and administering marijuana than I did. One of them even asked me to please keep him informed of how the Bureau of Narcotics responded to my request. "We'd be interested to know how they'd react to someone asking for marijuana for research," he said. That experience convinced me it would save time and effort to bypass NIMH entirely — a hunch that proved correct.

As things turned out, the Federal Bureau of Narcotics was the least unhelpful of all the bureaucracies involved. Much greater complications developed at the state government level in Massachusetts, and all of these problems became insignificant compared to opposition created by administrative personnel of both Harvard and Boston universities. It is not my purpose here to recount details of what became a frustrating bureaucratic battle, especially since those details would be embarrassing to the faculties of both institutions. What is relevant is simply the irrationality of the opposition, and it is relevant because it indicates the extent of bias in professions that like to regard themselves as free from bias. I will give one example.

Harvard Medical School (whose only control over the Boston University project was through me as a student) threatened to deny me academic credit for the work and thus prevent me from getting my medical degree if I gave marijuana to persons who had never had it before. Now, the use of "marijuana-naïve" subjects was an essential aspect of my experimental design because it was the only way to standardize set. Zinberg and I felt we were starting from scratch; no one had done what we were going to do — that is, try to find out what marijuana did on its own as distinct from what it did in the growing drug subculture. We reasoned that anyone who had tried marijuana had a definite set toward it that was beyond our control. But if we studied persons who had never tried the drug or seen it being used, and if we gave it to them in as neutral a setting as possible, we might isolate the purely pharmacological effects of marijuana. Harvard's Ad Hoc Committee on Human Studies did not agree. To quote from its report: "Eight of the eleven attending felt this was a major item and were concerned that the subjects introduced to the use of marijuana in the name of science might get 'hooked' on the drug."

It was clear that Harvard's real worries were of lawsuits and adverse publicity resulting from the experiments. After many deadlocks, the chairman of the committee, a well-known experimental physiologist, agreed to reconsider if a preliminary group of marijuana users survived the smoking of marijuana in our laboratory without disaster. Accordingly, we put five user subjects through our experimental procedures. The results were unexpected in that these people did just as well on a number of tests after smoking marijuana as they did when they were tested before smoking. (There were no disasters.) I wrote up a preliminary report of these experiments and took it to the Ad Hoc Committee chairman. He read it over, shook his head, and said, "Performed just as well after marijuana? The Committee isn't going to like this; this is going to look like a whitewash." In the end we just went ahead and gave marijuana to people who had never had it before (with their informed consent, of course) and never had any further communication with the committee. There were no catastrophes, and I got my degree.*

Because we encountered so many delays, the experiments were not finished until hours before I was due to start an internship in San Francisco. I began sorting out our results on the plane west. Zinberg departed for England as a visiting professor of social psychology at the London School of Economics, and Judith Nelsen, a Boston University graduate student who had worked with us, began the statistical analysis of our data. From Boston, London, and San Francisco, our final report took form. It was published in *Science* in December 1968 and generated an immense amount of international publicity (much to the consternation, I imagine, of a number of university committees). In retrospect, I think the most important result of our work was simply the demonstration that it was possible to administer marijuana to human volunteers in a laboratory, obtain usable results, and get away with it. A great many pessimists had tried their best to convince us that it was impossible — impossible to get marijuana, to get institutional support, to avoid legal repercussions, to avoid lawsuits, and so on and so on. We proved them wrong, and it was a satisfying victory.

But I do not pretend that our results provided any definitive answers to questions about marijuana. In fact, they stirred up a great deal of controversy.† Nor can I say that they very much influenced my own thinking about the drug. Most of what I am now going to

---

* It was amusing that, throughout this war with the Harvard bureaucracy, Zinberg and I had a difficult time finding marijuana-naïve subjects. It took two months of interviewing prospective volunteers to come up with nine men from the student population of Boston who had never tried marijuana.

† Here are our results, as summarized in our original *Science* article:
  1. It is feasible and safe to study the effects of marijuana on human volunteers who smoke it in a laboratory.
  2. In a neutral setting persons who are naïve to marijuana do not have strong subjective experiences after smoking low or high doses of the drug, and the effects they do

say about marijuana comes from my own experience with it, not from any laboratory studies I have conducted. Laboratory information is interesting and has its place, but I consider direct experience more important.

I will describe first the physical effects of marijuana, then the psychological effects. To begin with, I must stress the uniqueness of marijuana from the pharmacological point of view. It does not resemble any other known drug sufficiently to be classed with it. Its clinical actions are unique, and the chemicals it contains are unique in their molecular structure. Therefore, it is useful to regard marijuana as a class unto itself. And I consider it especially foolish to think of marijuana as a mild psychedelic, a label still being promoted by NIMH and the medical profession. Marijuana does not resemble the psychedelics, all of which are stimulants, even though it keeps company with them in the drug subculture. Calling it a mild psychedelic is tactically as well as factually foolish: I have met many persons who first tried psychedelics because they had been led to believe that LSD and mushrooms were bigger and better than marijuana, which they liked. Many first-time users

---

report are not the same as those described by regular users of marijuana who take the drug in the same neutral setting.

3. Marijuana-naïve persons do demonstrate impaired performance on simple intellectual and psychomotor tests after smoking marijuana; the impairment is dose-related in some cases.

4. Regular users of marijuana do get high after smoking marijuana in a neutral setting but do not show the same degree of impairment of performance on the tests as do naïve subjects. In some cases, their performance even appears to improve slightly after smoking marijuana.

5. Marijuana increases heart rate moderately.

6. No change in respiratory rate follows administration of marijuana by inhalation.

7. No change in pupil size occurs in short-term exposure to marijuana.

8. Marijuana administration causes dilatation of conjunctival blood vessels.

9. Marijuana treatment produces no change in blood-sugar levels.

10. In a neutral setting the physiological and psychological effects of a single, inhaled dose of marijuana appear to reach maximum intensity within one half-hour of inhalation, to be diminished after one hour, and to be completely dissipated by three hours. (A. T. Weil, N. E. Zinberg, J. M. Nelsen, "Clinical and Psychological Effects of Marijuana in Man," *Science* 162 [13 December 1968], p. 1234.)

of psychedelics are surprised — some of them unpleasantly — to find that these drugs are qualitatively different from pot.

In this section, I will use the term *marijuana* as a synonym for hemp drugs or cannabis. All preparations of hemp have similar effects, though they vary in potency. Potency is a measure of relative strength; it should not be confused with power, a measure of absolute strength, even though many physicians and drug experts ignore the distinction. For example, dextroamphetamine (Dexedrine) is about four times as potent a stimulant as amphetamine (Benzedrine), but if you take twenty milligrams of amphetamine, you will experience the same stimulation as if you had taken five milligrams of dextroamphetamine. By contrast, morphine is a more powerful pain reliever than aspirin: it produces qualitatively greater effects than aspirin regardless of dosage. Hashish, the concentrated resin of the hemp plant, is more potent than preparations of the whole plant (which are diluted by vegetable fiber) but no more powerful when equivalent doses are compared. Moreover, hashish as found in the United States is usually less potent than the most potent varieties of marijuana now available, probably because it deteriorates faster and takes longer to reach us. American users of hemp drugs use hashish and marijuana interchangeably; they regard government warnings about the greater dangers of hashish as further evidence that drug experts have little knowledge of the facts of drug use. Another myth propagated by government officials is that home-grown marijuana does not approach the potency of imported varieties. I have smoked samples of marijuana grown in Vermont, California, Oregon, and British Columbia that were as potent as the strongest Mexican or Colombian varieties I have come across. It is true that seeds of native hemp planted in their own environments produce fibrous plants with little resin, but seeds of imported plants, grown in many parts of the country, yield high-resin marijuana.

The acute (that is, short-term) physical effects of marijuana are easily discussed because there are so few of them. Marijuana causes a moderate increase in heart rate, reddening of the whites of the eyes, and drying of the mouth and eyes. No other clinically relevant effects have been documented, and it is unlikely that any will be. Of course, as pharmacologists look on finer and finer levels, they may find biochemical and other subcellular changes correlated with these acute clinical effects, but I would not consider them relevant to the experience of being high on the drug. And the unimpressiveness of these effects needs to be stressed: people who smoke marijuana are usually unaware of them. Dryness of the mouth is the most frequently noticed effect. Dryness of the eyes is usually apparent only to wearers of contact lenses. The increase in heart rate most often goes unnoticed, although it occasionally becomes the basis of a panic reaction in older, first-time users, who may interpret it to mean they are having a heart attack.

This virtual absence of effects on the body is most important because it underlines the disparity between the subjective and objective effects of the drug. One consequence of this disparity is that persons whose set toward the drug includes much anxiety (most first-time users, for example) can ignore the drug completely and pretend to themselves that nothing has happened. My Boston associates and I were repeatedly struck by this reaction in our marijuana-naïve subjects. They would sit in the laboratory with red eyes and heart rates of 130 beats per minute (normal resting pulse is 70 or 80) after smoking two large joints and would have no subjective responses at all. After the sessions, some of them would ask, "Did I have a drug tonight?" (We, of course, did not know for sure until the experiments were finished and the double-blind code was broken.) Very few drugs that trigger altered states of consciousness can be ignored so completely.

By contrast, alcohol, even in doses that trigger "social highs," begins to affect the nervous system in unmistakable ways. Slurring of speech and incoordination are apparent even to first-time users if they take enough. And it is this action on lower brain centers that accounts for the acute medical dangers of alcohol, which can lead to stupor, coma, and death from respiratory failure in doses not much higher than those leading to outright drunkenness. Conversely, the striking medical harmlessness of marijuana is correlated with its lack of clinically significant actions on the brain.

I believe this property of marijuana also accounts for its growing popularity as a recreational intoxicant among younger Americans, who have discovered the advantages of a high without a great deal of physiological distraction resulting from interference with the nervous system. Most persons I know who have switched to marijuana from alcohol (including many of my college and medical school classmates) have done so because they prefer the high; many are quite articulate about the drawbacks of using alcohol. The problem with alcohol, in addition to its greater pharmacological "noisiness," is that it is difficult to control. There is no question that alcohol can trigger a useful altered state of consciousness; a vast body of prose, poetry, and song from all ages testifies to its virtues. But in drinking, it is hard to maintain this state and terribly easy to cross over into a dose range where the pharmacological noise drowns out the high. When I drank in college, I invariably drank too much, no matter how often I told myself I would not. And the effects of too much alcohol make it difficult for me and many others to enjoy and make use of the high. Because marijuana is much quieter pharmacologically, the high is "purer," much more controllable, and much easier to maintain, even over a wide range of dosage. It is very hard to take too much marijuana by smoking (unless one has unusually potent material), and the consequence of too much is sedation rather than incapacitation. A marijuana high is also more subtle in that one must learn to notice it. For many persons, learning to be high on marijuana simply means unlearning a previous set — a process that has been called (not very accurately) "reverse tolerance." For all these reasons, I am inclined to agree with those who feel that marijuana gives a better high than alcohol, but for the same reasons I consider drugless highs better yet. (They are also still more subtle and require much more unlearning.)

If one eats marijuana or, especially, hashish, it is possible to experience an unpleasant overdose reaction or even a toxic psychosis, but toxic psychoses do not occur in response to smoking. This observation is one reason for thinking that hemp drugs have qualitatively different pharmacological effects when taken by mouth, probably because certain constituents of the resin are destroyed or changed by the heat of combustion. Chemical evidence is now coming in to support this idea that marijuana becomes noisier when eaten. Nevertheless, most ongoing government-sponsored research on marijuana is still using oral doses, making any results of questionable relevance to the world at large, where the drug is almost universally smoked.

Because marijuana is such an unimpressive pharmacological agent, it is not a very interesting drug to study in a laboratory. Pharmacologists cannot get a handle on it with their methods, and because they cannot see the reality of the nonmaterial state of consciousness that users experience, they are forced to design experimental situations very far removed from the real world in order to get measurable effects. There are three conditions under which marijuana can be shown to impair general psychological performance in laboratory subjects. They are: (1) by giving it to people who have never had it before; (2) by giving people very high doses that they are not used to (or giving it orally to people used to smoking it); and (3) by giving people very hard things to do, especially things that they have never had a chance to practice while under the influence of the drug. Under any of these three conditions, pharmacologists can demonstrate that marijuana impairs performance. And if we look at the work being done by government-funded researchers, all of it fulfills one or more of these conditions. In addition, the tests being used by these scientists are designed to look for impairments of functions that have nothing to do with why marijuana users put themselves in an altered state of consciousness. People who get high on marijuana do not sponta-neously try to do arithmetic problems or test their fine coordi-nation.

What pharmacologists cannot make sense of is that people who are high on marijuana cannot be shown, in objective terms, to be different from people who are not high. That is, if a marijuana user is allowed to smoke his usual doses and then to do things he has had a chance to practice while high, he does not appear to per-form any differently from someone who is not high. Now, this pat-tern of users performing better than nonusers is a general phe-nomenon associated with all psychoactive drugs. For example, an alcoholic will vastly outperform a nondrinker on any test if the two are equally intoxicated; he has learned to compensate for the ef-fects of the drug on his nervous system. But compensation can proceed only so far until it runs up against a ceiling imposed by the pharmacological action of the drug on lower brain centers. Again, since marijuana has no clinically significant action on lower brain centers, compensation can reach 100 percent with practice.

These considerations mean that there are no answers to ques-tions like, What does marijuana do to driving ability? The only pos-sible answer is, It depends. It depends on the person — whether he or she is a marijuana user, whether he or she has practiced driv-ing while under the influence of marijuana. In speaking to legisla-tive and medical groups, I have stated a personal reaction to this question in the form of the decision I would make if I were given the choice of riding with one of the following four drivers: (1) a person who had never smoked marijuana before and just had; (2) a marijuana smoker who had never driven while high and was just about to; (3) a high marijuana smoker who had practiced driving while high; and (4) a person with any amount of alcohol in him. I would unhesitatingly take driver number three as the best possi-ble risk. One may wonder how many drivers of types one and two are on our highways. Probably many. But there is some consola-tion in the fact that persons learning to do things under the influ-

ence of marijuana almost always are anxious about their performance and therefore tend to err on the side of overcaution.

The tendency for novice users of marijuana to imagine that
their psychological functioning is disrupted to a much greater degree than it actually is, is most noticeable in connection with subtle changes in speech. People who are high on marijuana seem to
have to do slightly more work than usual to remember from moment to moment the logical thread of what they are saying. This
change manifests itself in two ways: as a tendency to forget what
one started out to say, especially following an interruption, and a
tendency to go off on irrelevant tangents. Zinberg, Nelsen, and I
were able to pick up these changes in tape recordings of our
Boston subjects, but I must emphasize the adjective *subtle* in describing them. Someone not specially trained to listen for these
changes would not hear them. Interestingly enough, however,
marijuana users themselves often imagine they are not making
sense and become anxious about other people guessing that they
are high. Some users experience this subjective anxiety about
speech most intensely when they are talking on the telephone.
Here is a quote from such a user (a twenty-four-year-old male
medical student), which Zinberg and I included in a paper published in *Nature* in 1969:

> I've learned to do a lot of things when I'm stoned and seem to func-
> tion well in all spheres of activity. I can also "turn off" a high when
> that seems necessary. The one problem I have, however, is talking to
> straight people when I don't want them to know I'm stoned. It's re-
> ally scary because you constantly imagine you're talking nonsense
> and that the other person is going to realize you're high. That's never
> happened, though, so I conclude that I don't sound as crazy to others
> as I do to myself. It's worst on the telephone. Someone will call up
> and be talking to me, and when he stops I'll have no idea what he
> just said. Then I don't know what I'm supposed to answer and I have
> to stall until I get a clue as to what's expected of me. Again, even
> though this is very disconcerting, the other party never seems to no-

tice that anything's wrong unless he's a heavy pot smoker, too, and then it doesn't matter.[1]

Probably, the subtle difficulties in speech that high users pay great attention to are themselves manifestations of a change in a more general psychological function called immediate memory. It seems valid to distinguish three kinds of memory. The first has been termed immediate and seems to cover events of the past few seconds only. It is as if all information coming into the brain is held in some location for a very short time before a decision is made about where to store it. If it is to be filed in an accessible place, it passes to a second storage location called recent memory, where it may remain for days or, perhaps, weeks; otherwise it is salted away out of reach of ordinary consciousness. Eventually, if it is to be kept in an accessible place for a longer time, it moves to a third long-term storage location, which is the permanent memory file. Each of these locations has active connections to ordinary consciousness so that memories may be quickly retrieved from all of them in our normal waking state.

In senile dementia, the classic psychological change is loss of recent memory with sparing of immediate and long-term memory. Senile patients can remember strings of numbers read to them long enough to recite them back and can go into autobiographical detail about their childhoods. They cannot remember the date or the events of the previous day. By contrast, in certain forms of posttraumatic amnesia, immediate and recent memory are spared, but information filed prior to the trauma cannot be retrieved from the long-term memory storage. A person high on marijuana seems to have difficulty remembering what happened in the past few seconds, and the subtle speech changes reflect this difficulty. Furthermore, it looks as if a significant disturbance of immediate memory retrieval has few noticeable consequences in terms of behavior, although it may cause great anxiety in the mind of the person experiencing it.

This last observation raises an interesting question. Is the problem disturbance of immediate memory or anxiety about this change? Most people who have read the hypothesis Zinberg and I first presented in *Nature* have drawn the conclusion that marijuana interferes with immediate memory. In fact, the director of the National Institute of Mental Health, in testimony before Congress in 1970, used our results to support the statement that "more recent studies . . . in which researchers have learned some troublesome facts . . . make it impossible to give marijuana a clean bill of health."[2] I would once have gone along with this kind of reasoning, but the more I have thought about the matter, the more it has become clear to me that it is not useful to think of marijuana as interfering with one's awareness of the immediate past.

For one thing, disturbance of immediate memory seems to be a common feature of all altered states of consciousness in which attention is focused on the present. It can be noticed in hypnotic and other trances, meditation, mystic ecstasies, and highs associated with all drugs. Therefore, to call marijuana the cause of the phenomenon is probably unwise. In addition, the phrase *disturbance of immediate memory* bristles with negativity. Is it a negative description of a condition that might just as well be looked at positively? I believe so. In fact, the ability to live entirely in the present, without paying attention to the immediate past or future, is precisely the goal of meditation and the exact aim of many religious disciplines. The rationale behind living in the present is stated in ancient Hindu writings and forms a prominent theme of Buddhist and Christian philosophy as well: to the extent that consciousness is diverted into the past and future — both of which are unreal — to that extent is it unavailable for use in the real here and now. Consequently, monastic systems of all faiths have used devices like gongs and bells to focus the consciousness of the novice on the immediate reality of the present, and contemporary instructional materials on mental and spiritual development stress the same theme. Here are a few examples:

1. From *A Practical Guide to Yoga* by James Hewitt:

When the mind is stilled by Raja Yoga, time — that is to say, *psychological* time — ceases to exist. For time is relative. It only exists when one thing is taken in relation to another. If I go on a train journey my leaving the train at my destination, taken in relation to my getting in, shows a passage of time. Similarly, if I think of "fruit," and in a split second follow with another thought "apples," time has passed, and I am aware of its passing. But if the mind takes one thought and holds it, one-pointed and still, time is erased; it ceases — psychologically — to exist.

In the hurly-burly of civilized living we rarely find time, or even give a thought to living in the NOW. We spend our NOW thinking of the past or dreaming of the future. Raja Yoga enables us to be still and experience eternity, as defined by Boethius: "to hold and possess the whole fullness of life in one moment, here and now, past and present and to come."[3]

2. The following excerpt is from C. S. Lewis' *The Screwtape Letters* — a witty and practical statement of orthodox Christian theology cast in the form of letters from a senior devil, Screwtape, to a junior devil, Wormwood, who is trying to capture the soul of an earthly "patient":

My Dear Wormwood,
    I had noticed, of course, that the humans were having a lull in their European war [World War II] — what they naively call "The War!" — and am not surprised that there is a corresponding lull in the patient's anxieties. Do we want to encourage this or to keep him worried? Tortured fear and stupid confidence are both desirable states of mind. Our choice between them raises important questions.
    The humans live in time, but our Enemy destines them to eternity. He therefore, I believe, wants them to attend chiefly to two things, to eternity itself and to that point of time which they call the Present. For the Present is the point at which time touches eternity.

Of the present moment, and of it only, humans have an experience analogous to the experience which our Enemy has of reality as a whole; in it alone freedom and actuality are offered them. He would therefore have them continually concerned either with eternity (which means being concerned with Him) or with the Present — either meditating on their eternal union with, or separation from, Himself, or else obeying the present voice of conscience, bearing the present cross, receiving the present grace, giving thanks for the present pleasure.

Our business is to get them away from the eternal and from the Present.[4]

3. From *Concentration and Meditation* by Christmas Humphreys:

As the sequence of day and night, so is the alternation of work and rest, and it is in these minutes of comparative repose that the difference appears between the trained and the untrained student of mind-development. The beginner allows his energy to drain away in idle conversation or mental rambling, in vague revision of past experiences or anxiety over events as yet unborn, or in a thousand other wasteful ways for which, were he spending gold instead of mental energy, he would be hailed as a reckless spendthrift to be avoided by all prudent men.[5]

4. The following summary of J. Krishnamurti's philosophy of time is from *Metaphysical Approach to Reality* by Ganga Sahai. Mr. Krishnamurti's books are widely available in the West.

There is a state of being which Krishnamurti calls the timeless. It comes with the realization that the only real moment is the moment of the Now, the eternal present; the past and future taken as "no-more" and "not-yet" are illusions.

The center, the observer, is memory. The center is always in the past. Therefore, the center is not a living thing. It is a memory of what has been. When there is complete attention, there is no observer . . .

Life is broken up and this breaking of life, caused by the center "me," is time. If we look at the whole of existence without the center "me" there is no time.

The new dimension is the silent mind. It is always in the present, always in the Now. It is the timeless mind that really exists.[6]

Thus the pharmacological way of thinking leads to the formulation of a hypothesis built upon an incorrect causal attribution and a negatively biased description of a phenomenon assigned great value in other ways of thinking. The pharmacologist says marijuana interferes with immediate memory, and by using tests in which one is penalized for not paying full attention to the past, the pharmacologist can produce evidence to document his hypothesis. The federal government supports this kind of research with money appropriated by Congress. It does not fund research designed to look for the positive advantages of having one's full awareness focused on the present.

In a similar way, all other psychological effects of marijuana turn out to be common features of altered states of consciousness unassociated with drugs, and whenever pharmacology describes them in negative ways, it is possible to look at them positively from the point of view of conscious experience. The perceptual changes reported by marijuana users are another example. Here again is an apparent paradox since all testing to date has failed to show any objective changes in sensory function during acute marijuana intoxication. If pharmacologists paid closer attention to what users say, they would find their way out of this paradox. There is no indication from persons high on marijuana that their sense organs are working differently than usual. Rather, the change seems to be in what they do with incoming sensory information. For instance, many users claim that listening to music is more interesting and pleasurable when they are high. They do not claim that they hear tones of lower volume or that they can better discriminate between pitches of tones. Yet all of the testing of auditory function under marijuana has been aimed at the ear — at auditory thresholds, pitch discrimination, and the like.

In 1969, when I still thought as a pharmacologist in my professional life, I wrote the following paragraph in an article, "Cannabis," published in England in *Science Journal:*

> It would make more sense to look for effects not on the ear but rather on that part of the brain that processes auditory information. Cannabis seems to affect the secondary perception of sensory information, not the primary reception of it. Unfortunately, it is considerably harder to study secondary perception because the neural organization underlying it is less accessible to direct experimentation and much less well understood. A working hypothesis is that incoming sensory information (such as auditory signals representing music) normally follows conditioned pathways through the secondary perception network in order to get to consciousness. Under Cannabis, which might interfere with this normal processing, information may take novel routes to consciousness and thus be perceived in novel ways. Such a model would explain why users often say that under Cannabis they see things for the first time "as they really are," or why they dwell on aspects of complex visual or auditory stimuli they would ordinarily ignore.[7]

I now realize that altered secondary perception of sensory information is intrinsic to all altered states of consciousness, whether triggered by drugs or not. Therefore, it no longer seems profitable to me to try to understand how marijuana "causes" the effect. In addition, I no longer subscribe to the negative hypothesis that marijuana interferes with normal processing of perceptual data. Rather, I observe that in altered states of consciousness, people frequently gain the ability to interpret their perceptions in new ways and that this ability seems to be the key to freedom from bondage to the senses. For example, hypnotic anesthesia is nothing more than another way of perceiving pain. Patients, fully aware but in a state of focused consciousness, learn the "trick" of separating the pain itself from their reactions to it. They are thus free to perceive the pain in a novel way — something going on "out there" but not hurting. (One hypnotist I know produces this state with the suggestion that "the hurt is going out of the pain.")

Furthermore, the ability to produce anesthesia at will (a power frequently demonstrated by adepts at yoga) may be no more than a trifling use of this freedom to experience sensations in other ways. Once you learn the process, you may become aware of many more useful things to do with it than ignore pain. For example, the conscious experience of unity behind the diversity of phenomena — said by sages and mystics of all centuries to be the most blissful and uplifting of human experiences — may require nothing more than a moment's freedom to stand back from the inrush of sensory information and look at it in a different way than usual.

If all the so-called psychological effects of marijuana are really not attributable to marijuana, and if the physical effects that are attributable to it are so unimpressive, what, then, is marijuana? To my mind, the best term for marijuana is *active placebo* — that is, a substance whose apparent effects on the mind are actually placebo effects in response to minimal physiological action. Pharmacologists sometimes use active placebos (in contrast to inactive placebos like sugar pills) in drug testing; for example, niacin, which causes warmth and flushing, has been compared with LSD in some laboratory experiments. But pharmacologists do not understand that all psychoactive drugs are really active placebos since the psychic effects arise from consciousness, elicited by set and setting, in response to physiological cues.

Thus, for most marijuana users, the occasion of smoking a joint becomes an opportunity or excuse for experiencing a mode of consciousness that is available to everyone all the time, even though many people do not know how to get high without using a drug. Not surprisingly, regular marijuana users often find themselves becoming high spontaneously. (The pharmacologist invokes "residual concentrations of Cannabis constituents in the body" to explain this observation.) The user who correctly interprets the significance of spontaneous highs takes the first step away from dependence on the drug to achieve the desired state of consciousness and the first step toward freer use of the nervous system. All drugs that seem to give highs behave this way; all are active placebos. But the less physiological noise, the easier it is for a user to understand the true nature of drugs and their highly indirect relationship to states of consciousness. Alcohol users are less likely to find themselves spontaneously high because they have come to think that "high" includes all the pharmacological noise of alcohol. At the same time, marijuana, while providing a better opportunity to make the jump to drugless highs, is more insidious as a creator of illusion, for it enables users to pretend that they are not really dependent on it at the same time that it reinforces the notion that highs come in joints, an irony that recalls another unsettling comment of C. S. Lewis's Screwtape: "Nowhere do we tempt so successfully as on the very steps of the altar."[8]

5. Clues from the Amazon

I T WAS IMPOSSIBLE TO WORK in the Harvard Botanical Museum and not develop a powerful longing to see the Amazon. The New World tropics, aside from their beauty and energy, are the richest source of psychoactive plants in the world. Some species are still unidentified botanically. And the Indians of the Amazon basin use more drugs of plant origin than any other peoples.

In the summer of 1965, after completing my first year of medical school, I flew to Bogotá and thence to Leticia, Colombia's tiny port on the Amazon, a quaint town midway between the two large cities of the upper river: Manaus in Brazil and Iquitos in Peru. Along with a graduate student of Richard Schultes I was to collect a large quantity of the leaves of a particular tree that grew in the secondary forest around Leticia; it was a member of the coffee family — a botanical group rich in alkaloids that includes such species as ipecac (the source of emetine) and cinchona (the source of quinine). I do not pretend that my experience in this part of the world is extensive; in fact, half of my summer was spent in the Andes, far above the dense forests. Also, I paid more attention to the ubiquitous chewing of coca leaf (the source of cocaine) in the Bolivian highlands than to the ritual use of psychedelic plants by forest tribes, and my interests at the time centered on the pharmacology of psychoactive plants rather than on the experiences they triggered. Nevertheless, this visit gave me a chance to make some observations and learn some facts that struck me as noteworthy even though I did not fully understand their significance. Now, as I have come to think about drugs from the point of view of consciousness, the importance of this information is clear to me.

Simply put, there exist in the Amazonian regions societies that make liberal use of drugs to alter awareness but do not appear to have problems with them. The tastes of these tribes run to stimulants and, especially, psychedelics rather than to sedative-hypnotics or narcotics, and they have available to them a jungleful of potential intoxicants. Schultes has written:

> It is of interest that the New World is very much richer in narcotic* plants than the Old and that the New World boasts at least 40 species of hallucinogens as opposed to half a dozen species native to the Old World . . . There is a real need for more field studies of narcotic plants in the New World. If we are to delve into the few remaining virgin areas of aboriginal American life before they are forever blotted out by encroaching civilization, we must train men in interdisciplinary fields, especially in the overlapping phases of anthropology, botany, chemistry, and the pharmaceutical sciences.[1]

The far greater prevalence of hallucinogenic plants in the New World than in the Old — a mystifying difference from the point of view of botany — can be explained by the present theory of consciousness, as I shall show at the end of this chapter. What is most relevant about all these plants is that they are natural sources of some of the very drugs that are associated with problems in our society. For example, in the summer of 1967, a scientific expedition to the Rio Negro in northwesternmost Brazil observed the use of an intoxicating snuff called *epená* by a tribe of Waiká Indians in the tiny jungle village of Maturacá. Schultes, who participated in the expedition, and Holmstedt, a Swedish toxicologist, wrote of this tribe: "The Maturacá Waiká store *epená* in a large bamboo tube hanging from the house beams, and it is employed by any adult male singly or in groups at any time as well as during festivals. The tube is kept full, and the snuff, consequently, is always available for use. Every now and then, an Indian will take the snuff, become intoxicated, dance and sing, all alone with the rest

* In botanical (as opposed to medical) usage, *narcotic* is synonymous with "intoxicating."

of the village going about its usual chores and not paying any heed to him."[2] The principal ingredient of this snuff is the blood-red resin of a tree of the nutmeg family. In 1969, a group of Swedish chemists, including Holmstedt, reported that the resin contains large amounts of DMT and related psychedelics. DMT (dimethyltryptamine) has been available in synthetic form on the American black market. It is snuffed, smoked (usually by mixing the crystals with tobacco, marijuana, or mint leaves), or (rarely) injected and is very similar to LSD in its pharmacological effects except that its duration of action is less than thirty minutes (compared to ten or twelve hours for LSD). Because it is so short-acting, the American drug subculture nicknamed it the "businessman's high."

When I say that Amazonian Indians have no problems with drugs like DMT, I mean that people in these societies do not take these drugs to rebel against parents or teachers, to drop out of the social process, or to hurt themselves. Neither is their drug use in any way linked with antisocial patterns of behavior. And since the drugs, in many cases, are the same ones tied to antisocial patterns of use in the United States, the differences cannot have much basis in pharmacology. What, then, are these Indians doing differently that enables them to live with drugs and not suffer the negative consequences of drug use?

Conventional scholarship does not help us answer this question because it has never asked it. Although the drug use of South American Indians has been looked at by anthropologists, botanists, and pharmacologists, it has never been studied by anyone interested primarily in alteration of consciousness. Nor has anyone visited these tribes with the express purpose of finding out why they fare better than we do in their relationships with substances that trigger altered states of consciousness.

From my own studies, readings, and observations, I have come to feel that the success of Indian tribes in this regard has to do with the ways they think about drugs and states of consciousness and with certain principles of drug use they have discovered. Above all, they admit to themselves that their world contains many substances that can give access to altered states of consciousness. They do not try to eradicate the substances or prevent people from having access to them. This attitude strikes me as highly realistic in view of the abundance of hallucinogenic plants in the forest. Moreover, nature still dominates man in the New World tropics, and one does not simply make unwanted manifestations of nature go away. Vegetable life grows so fast on this part of the planet that a cleared area is overgrown again in a few weeks if not constantly tended. The Indians who live in this plant-dominated world wisely choose not to fight nature's tendency to shower them with psychoactive plants. Instead, they have explored the alternative of trying to make these plants work for them — to incorporate their use into society in beneficial ways.

I consider it most significant that these Indians use drugs in natural forms. They often prepare natural substances in elaborate ways; for example, the resin that goes into *epená* is concentrated by boiling and mixed with inert ingredients to produce the final snuff. But they do not attempt to refine these substances into pure, potent forms or to extract active principles from psychoactive plants. By contrast, most of the drugs in use in our society — aside from wine and beer, caffeine beverages, tobacco, marijuana, and occasional peyote — are highly refined, often synthetic chemicals.

It is a striking empirical fact that the difficulties individuals and societies get into with drugs appear to correlate with the purity or potency of substances in use: the more potent the drugs, the more trouble associated with them. Opium forms a relatively harmless habit in that a high percentage of users can take it for years without developing troublesome problems with tolerance. Dependence on opium, if stable, can be as consistent with social productivity as dependence on coffee or tobacco. But when morphine, the active principle of opium, is isolated and made available, problems appear. In particular, a significant percentage of users (though possibly still a minority) finds it impossible to achieve equilibrium with habitual use of morphine or with the still more potent derivative, heroin, and these unstable users eventually behave in socially disruptive ways. The same kinds of comparisons can be made between coca leaf and cocaine. In all cases, the more potent forms are associated with more problems. The same trend is obvious in comparisons of societies that use different forms of alcohol. The kinds of alcoholism are worse and the numbers of people affected greater in countries like Finland and Sweden where distilled liquors are preferred than in countries like Italy where wine and beer predominate.

In addition, there is great logic behind the supposition that natural forms of drugs are inherently less dangerous than derived products. Plants that trigger altered states of consciousness never contain just one chemical. Usually, they contain a host of related compounds, all of which contribute to the pharmacological action of the whole plant. Opium, for example, contains twenty-one alkaloids besides morphine. Peyote has more than a score of alkaloids of which mescaline is just one. Now, it is true that one compound can often be identified as the principal constituent in that it reproduces most of the action of the whole plant, but it seems to me a most unhelpful way of thinking to call this compound the active principle and to dismiss all the rest as inactive. It is also true that the other compounds may do little when administered to subjects in isolated fashion. (For example, the inactive alkaloids of peyote may cause nothing more than nausea and dizziness if taken in pure form.) But this observation does not mean that these other constituents are inactive in the whole plant. Their action is to modify the action of the dominant constituent: to play down some of its effects, to enhance others, much as harmonic overtones modify the sound of a pure tone to produce the distinctive timbre of a musical instrument. Ethyl butyrate, the pure chemical ester that is the principal component of artificial strawberry flavoring, could be described as the active principle of that fruit, but to my mind there is a world of difference between it and the natural taste of strawberries.

Yet modern pharmacologists work on the assumption that pure

active principles are equivalent to complex natural drugs. Thus they study cocaine instead of coca, mescaline instead of peyote, psilocybin instead of magic mushrooms, and now THC (tetrahydrocannabinol) instead of marijuana. During our marijuana experiments in Boston, Norman Zinberg and I were under pressure by pharmacologists to use THC rather than marijuana to make our studies more "meaningful." And much of the research now being funded by the government is using pure THC (often administered orally) rather than the natural drug. Pharmacologists cling to this way of thinking because they imagine pure compounds give better results. What they mean is that laboratory studies can be designed more rigorously if one administers exact doses of single compounds. But if experimental rigor is obtained at the expense of relevance to the world beyond the laboratory, it is not desirable. People do not eat THC outside of laboratories; they smoke marijuana. The subjective experience of smoking marijuana is not the same as the subjective experience of eating (or smoking) THC. Similarly, mescaline is not peyote, cocaine is not coca,* morphine is not opium. And, in view of the observation that potent derivatives cause far more trouble to human beings than natural forms of drugs, these differences seem very much worth respecting. I have already mentioned the symmetries in thinking one can see

* "... the effects of coca leaf often have been presumed to be embodied in the alkaloid cocaine, albeit in a more potent form, with the result that the majority of the physiological research for the last 50 years has been performed solely with cocaine and not with other preparations of coca leaves. However, many physicians have emphasized that the effects of these two are not identical, and particularly that the therapeutic qualities of coca are not represented completely in the active principle cocaine. An important conclusion in this regard is that active principles and particularly alkaloids can exert quite different effects when administered as they are naturally combined in the plant than when administered singly in pure form. Very little is known about the physiological activity of the associate alkaloids of the coca plant, and still less about their effects in combination. The necessity of looking into the possible importance of these other compounds is emphasized by the fact that an Indian will frequently reject the bitter coca leaves with the highest percentage of cocaine in favor of the sweeter leaves which are richer in the more aromatic alkaloids." (R. T. Martin, "The Role of Coca in the History, Religion, and Medicine of South American Indians," Economic Botany 24:4, 1970, p. 436.)

between drug abusers and drug researchers; I think it is no accident that both groups in our society prefer to use pure, potent chemicals rather than substances in the forms given to us by nature. And I consider the Indians' preference for natural drugs one reason why they do not have a drug problem.

Another reason, perhaps a more important one, is that they recognize the normality of the human drive to experience altered states of consciousness periodically and the prominence of the drive in growing children. Rather than try to thwart the expression of this need, the Indians choose to introduce children to these experiences by letting them try drugs under supervision. Supervision is provided by the tribal expert in such matters, usually the shaman. It is noteworthy that shamans are drug experts solely by virtue of their own experience; because of their familiarity with states of consciousness induced by drugs they are considered qualified to guide others through these experiences.

Furthermore, the use of drugs in Indian societies is highly ritualized. That is, drugs are taken in certain ways for certain purposes. Some drugs are used only by shamans for purposes of divination or diagnosing of illness. For example, the shaman might take a drug and sit with his patient; while in an altered state of consciousness, he would attempt to commune with the spirit world in order to learn the nature of the disease. Other drugs, like the *ayahuasca* of certain Peruvian tribes, are used by adolescent males in coming-of-age rites. Still others, like the *epená* of the Waiká, are used as recreational intoxicants, and recreation is recognized as a legitimate purpose for altering consciousness. All of these uses are surrounded by ritual: at every step of the process, from cutting the plants to administering the prepared drugs, the Indians do things in traditional, careful, often elaborate ways, even when use appears to be casual, as in the case of the Waikás and their *epená* snuff.

Here, for example, is a description by a Peruvian youth who was captured by Amahuaca Indians of the preparation of *ayahuasca* by the tribal medicine man. The Amahuaca made this powerful hal-

lucinogenic drink (also known as *yagé* and *caapi*) from the thick
stems of a woody vine (*Banisteriopsis caapi*) and the leaves of a
shrub (probably *Diplopterys cabrerana*):

> ... the serious preparations started, accompanied by almost contin-
> uous chanting. First the vine was cut into one-foot pieces with the
> stone ax and pounded on a flat stone with a large wooden mallet un-
> til it was well mashed.
>
> The old man chanted:
>
> > "*Nixi honi* [i.e., vine whose extract produces visions]
> > vision vine
> > boding spirit of the forest
> > origin of our understanding give up your magic power
> > to our potion
> > illuminate our mind
> > bring us foresight
> > show us the designs of our enemies
> > expand our knowledge
> > expand our understanding
> > of our forest."
>
> A layer of mashed vine pieces was then carefully arranged in the bot-
> tom of a large new clay pot. On top of this was laid a layer of the
> leaves in the shape of a fan. And as he did this [he] chanted:
>
> > "Bush with markings of the serpent
> > give us your leaves
> > for our potion
> > bring us favor
> > of the boa
> > source of good fortune."
>
> Then alternating layers of mashed vine and leaves were put in
> place until the pot was more than half full. Clear water from the
> stream was then added until the plant material was well covered.
>
> A slow fire was started under the pot and the cooking was main-
> tained at a very low simmer for many hours until the liquid was re-
> duced to less than half.

When the cooking process was completed the fire was removed and, after cooling, the plant material was withdrawn from the liquid. After several hours of further cooling and settling, the clear green liquid was carefully dipped off into small clay pots, each fitted with a tight cover.

The entire process took three days, being done with utter calmness and deliberation. The interminable chants accompanied each step, invoking the spirits of the vine, the shrub, and the other forest spirits.

This carefully and reverently prepared extract provided the potion for many subsequent *ayahuasca* sessions in the peaceful and secluded forest glade, sessions that progressed to incredible vision fantasies.[3]

This kind of ritual seems to protect individuals and groups from the negative effects of drugs, possibly by establishing a framework of order around their use. At least, people who use drugs ritually tend not to get into trouble with them, whereas people who abandon ritual and use drugs wantonly tend to have problems. We can see this protective function of ritual in our own society with our uses of alcohol. Americans who lay down a ritual for drinking — for example, people who drink only after 6 P.M., only with others present, only with food present, and only for a specified period before supper for the purpose of promoting social intercourse — are not the people who get into trouble with alcohol. Americans who get into trouble with alcohol are those who begin to use it without ritualistic rules and forms; uncontained by ritual, their drug use becomes unstable and begins to disrupt their lives.

I see the same principle at work among people I know who use marijuana. Those who use it ritually — that is, in groups as a recreational intoxicant or before going to a movie or before eating a good meal — do not have their lives taken over by their drug use. But those who dispense with ritual and smoke marijuana whenever they feel like it begin to get into worse and worse relationships with the drug. I remember also that when I lived and worked in the Haight-Ashbury district of San Francisco, the people I met who were in the very worst relationships with drugs (usually with methamphetamine, barbiturates, alcohol, and heroin) were always the people who had done away with rules entirely and used drugs according to no logical plan.

Probably, the effectiveness of ritual is independent of its content. I do not think it matters much what rules one makes for using drugs as long as one makes rules. If a rationale is needed for these rules, any rationale will do as long as it is consistent with prevailing beliefs. In Indian societies ritual is often explained in terms of respect for the god or spirit supposed to dwell within the magic plant. In American society, ritual may be understood as "good social form." In either case, the principle works to protect users from the negative potential of drugs.

One aspect of Indian ritual that deserves special emphasis is the use of altered states of consciousness for positive ends. That is, drug-induced states are not entered for negative reasons (such as escape from boredom or anxiety); rather, they are entered because they can be of positive usefulness to individuals and the tribe. I stress this point because it contrasts sharply with practices in the United States. Very many Americans take drugs for negative reasons or no reasons at all, and, again, I suspect this difference is a key factor in our having a drug problem. The principle that positive application of altered consciousness is protective is apparent among amphetamine users in our country. People who take amphetamines in order to use the stimulation for positive ends — for example, students who take them only to study for exams — do not tend to get into trouble with stimulants. The people who do get into trouble with amphetamines are those who begin to take them just because they like the feeling of stimulation. Just liking the feelings drugs provide without using those feelings for positive purposes seems to me to be the beginning of most bad relationships with drugs — that is, patterns of use destined to become more and more unstable and more and more dominating of the user's life.

This principle should be intuitively obvious because drug experiences are rarely pleasant when one's set is couched in negative terms. The person who expects a joint of marijuana or a tab of acid to undo a preexisting depression often has the drug backfire by intensifying the negative mental state. I have seen this pattern again and again among users of all drugs in this country and have experienced it myself. On every occasion that I have smoked marijuana or taken a psychedelic out of boredom or in order to escape depression, I have experienced exactly the opposite result. Consequently, when patients or friends ask my advice about trying drugs like marijuana or psychedelics for the first time, I urge them not to do so unless they can phrase their expectations in positive terms.

These observations are further evidence that the "magic" of drugs resides within the mind of the user, not in the drugs — a principle the Indians do not seem to have grasped. Most tribes that alter consciousness by chemical means protect themselves from this disruptive potential of drugs by using natural substances, by educating children in their "right" use, by surrounding the process with ritual, and by applying the altered states of consciousness to positive ends for the general welfare. But they tend not to realize that the experiences can be had without the drugs. Rather, they consider the plant sources of their intoxicants magical — the dwelling places of gods or spirits that transport the user to divine realms when they enter the body. Consistent with this view is the tendency of Indians to use drugs that produce considerable pharmacological noise. *Ayahuasca, epená,* and, certainly, the peyote of North American Indians all have powerful effects on the physical nervous system. In Indian societies, set and setting strongly encourage individuals to interpret these effects as preludes to intense, desired states of consciousness. By contrast, non-Indians who try these drugs, even in the same settings, often experience these same effects as symptoms of physical illness.

Set is so important that it can lead people to use as cues for positive experiences sensations that would otherwise be experienced in very negative ways. It is hard to see this principle at work in our country today because most people have definite sets toward psychedelics. But in 1960, when a number of Americans had never heard of LSD, it was possible to see what this drug did in people who expected nothing of it. I knew of a few cases in that year in which LSD was administered to people without their knowledge. When they experienced the stimulation and perceptual changes directly caused by the drug, they interpreted these sensations as the onset of physical illness (such as food poisoning); they did not use them as opportunities to enter desirable altered states of consciousness.

Here, I think, is an explanation for the prevalence of hallucinogenic plants in the New World. Schultes has written:

> ... whether because of cultural differences or floristic peculiarities or for some other as yet unappreciated reason, the New World is much richer in narcotic plants than the Old. These statistics, naturally, relate merely to those plants the narcotic properties of which man has discovered in his trial and error experimentation during the course of human history. The longer I consider this question, the more I am convinced that there may exist in the world's flora an appreciable number of such plants not yet uncovered by the experimenting natives and still to be found by the enquiring phytochemist.[4]

It is my belief that there are just as many plants in the Old World that do things to you (that is, can serve as active placebos); New World Indians are set to interpret the changes in a particular way. If Amazonian natives could be transplanted to the tropical regions of Africa, I would predict that they would soon discover a great array of new magic plants in the Old World and would learn to use them just as sensibly. It would be good to know much more about the general attitudes of these most interesting people, especially since their culture is about to disappear. I plan to return to South America in the very near future in order to try to understand them better.

Later on I shall suggest ways our society can change in order to move toward the Indian model of socially beneficial drug use without abuse. Here, I am still concerned with questions of individual behavior, and I would like to point out the relevance of the Indian model to the individual's use of drugs. If one decides to use drugs as the primary method of altering consciousness, one would be wise to imitate Indians in four ways:

1. Use natural drugs in natural ways.

It is good to learn to prefer natural drugs to synthetic or refined ones, less potent ones to more potent ones. The person who is intensely curious about narcotics would be better off experimenting with opium than with heroin. It is better to be involved with coca leaf than with cocaine. Getting high on beer and wine is healthier than getting high on spirits.

Moreover, it is wise to introduce drugs into the body in natural ways. Intravenous injection of any chemical is such an unnatural route of administration that, to my mind, it is an unreasonable practice even on a one-shot basis, let alone a habitual one. People who shoot drugs like heroin and cocaine may well be using compounds that are less dangerous medically than alcohol, but their habits are probably worse than those of excessive drinkers; taking drugs by mouth is much to be preferred to injecting them in veins (or inhaling them into lungs).

My strong feelings about intravenous use of drugs do not arise from any moral sentiments. Rather, it seems to be that we are not born with direct access to our veins for very good reasons that are understood but not applied by clinical pharmacologists. It is well known that the response of a person to a drug with general effects on the nervous system is more directly related to the rate of increase of concentration in the bloodstream and brain than to the absolute dose. Now, when one injects a drug directly into a vein, it is possible to increase blood and brain levels very fast. The toxicity of drugs and their addictiveness over time also correlate with their rates of increase of concentration in the blood and brain.

The directness of intravenous injection is obvious. It may be less obvious that inhaling and smoking are even more efficient — and therefore dangerous — ways of putting drugs into the body, but this is the case. With injection a drug is diluted in a relatively large volume of venous blood, must go to the heart, thence to the lungs and back to the heart before being pumped to the brain. When drugs like nicotine, cocaine, and methamphetamine are smoked and inhaled deeply, they go from lungs to heart to brain in one pass and undergo less dilution in relatively smaller volumes of arterial blood. Taking drugs by inhalation is one step removed from injecting them directly into the brain. For this reason, drug smoking is associated with the most stubborn forms of addiction.

These facts are well illustrated by the different patterns of use people establish with coca leaves and their derivatives. Indians who chew the whole leaves do not experience tolerance or toxicity and generally do not become dependent. People who snort refined cocaine often get into trouble with it if they have regular access to the drug. They experience physical and, especially, behavioral toxicity and have great difficulty limiting use. Those who inject cocaine become fascinated with the brief, intense "rush" of stimulation and euphoria; they are even more likely to become dependent users and to suffer adverse effects. Crackheads — those who smoke a pure form of cocaine — get the most intense effects of all and show the highest incidence of toxicity and addiction. The subjective experience of a drug taken by injection or inhalation is more extreme than the experience of the same drug taken orally, at least in those components of the experience directly related to changes in the physical nervous system. In practice, this means that the physiological noise associated with highs comes on much more dramatically when drugs are injected or smoked, just as it is much more intense (or, better, less muted) when potent derivatives are used rather than natural substances. Therefore, less natural drugs used in less natural ways tend to reinforce the materialistic illusion and reduce the probability of recognition of spontaneous natural highs. Until one notices one's own spontaneous highs, one cannot begin to develop them. The more natural the means used to trigger highs, the more likely that one will eventually experience highs unassociated with any material triggers. This goal is the aim of yoga and many other systems.

2. Use drugs ritually.

The tendency of habitual drug use to disrupt one's life can be contained by using drugs according to self-made rules. It does not matter what the rules are as long as they are acceptable and consistent with other beliefs. Such rules might concern times and places for using drugs and should define the purposes for which drugs are taken.

3. Seek advice from people who *know* what they are talking about.

The best guidance in the use of drugs comes from analogs of shamans — that is, from people qualified by virtue of their own experience. Of course, drug experience in itself does not necessarily confer this kind of authority. But academic degrees and memberships in professional societies by themselves certainly do not confer it.

In the midst of our emotional turmoil about the drug problem, many of us fail to notice that most of the authorities who are supported by public funds, quoted extensively in the scientific and lay press, and sought out for advice by policy makers have never themselves experienced highs in association with drugs or, if they have, keep that knowledge secret and do not draw upon it for answers to the problems they wish to solve. In February 1970, for example, at a government-sponsored symposium in California of noted drug experts, I listened to one of NIMH's star marijuana researchers brag to other participants that he was "a virgin with respect to pot and intend to keep it that way." A supreme irony of the American drug problem is the bias promulgated by the professional community that scientists who have used drugs have necessarily lost their objectivity and thus are disqualified from giving information on the subject. This kind of thinking leads us to ignore the only sources of the information we need to begin to change things for the better.

4. Use drugs for positive reasons.

I have repeatedly stated that there are more and less useful ways of interpreting our perceptions. My own experience is that we have greater access to the more useful varieties when we are in states of consciousness other than the ordinary waking state, which indicates that there is an important choice to be made between different kinds of thinking. I would like now to focus attention on that difference.

6. The Solar Mind: Straight Thinking

I N THE FIRST CHAPTER I wrote that I "do not have any special case to make for or against the use of drugs." It may have occurred to some readers, however, that I seem to have a case to make for something. And so I do. While I am not for or against the use of drugs, I make no secret of my belief that it is good to learn to spend time consciously in states of consciousness other than the ordinary waking state. In fact, this bias underlies much of what I have written up to now. Earlier I made no effort to justify this point of view except to note occasional examples of the positive implications of consciousness alteration (such as the possibility of voluntary control of the autonomic nervous system). Now I wish to give a formal explanation. The essence of what I have to say is simply this: altered states of consciousness, consciously entered, seem to me to be doors to using the mind in ways that are better than those most of us follow most of the time. I will use the term *deep* to designate these better ways and the term *straight* to designate the ordinary ways.

The metaphor of the sun and moon is also useful to represent these two aspects of the mind. Solar mind is ordinary mind, in which straight thinking predominates. Lunar mind reveals itself only when the sun sets, when ordinary consciousness is stilled. It is then we can experience deep thinking.

I am well aware that some of these terms have many meanings far removed from the specific ones intended here. *Straight* can mean "honest," "not curved," "not homosexual," or even (in the subcultural slang of previous generations) "in possession of illegal drugs." To many people *deep* simply denotes "profound." I will try to make these words work for the different ways of thinking I want to describe. Other terms have been suggested to me ("unenlightened" vs. "enlightened"; "linear" vs. "nonlinear"; "rational" vs. "nonrational"), but they seem to me cumbersome and less natural. I will continue to talk about straight thinking and deep thinking and request the reader to regard these as technical terms with particular definitions, to be explained in this chapter and the next.

The relative merit of straight versus deep thinking is by far the most important of all the garbled issues of the drug controversy, and also the most anxiety-provoking. The anxiety arises entirely from ego-centered consciousness because it concerns the deeply felt issue of self-esteem. When people who use drugs claim to have reached higher levels of consciousness or greater awareness, they automatically produce negative thoughts of lower levels of consciousness and lesser awareness in people who do not use drugs. Thus, these groups become polarized and begin to fight with each other symbolically, ritually, or even physically. When people are fighting they often fail to notice what is most important, such as evidence that higher levels of consciousness exist and are available to all of us.

If we can detach ourselves from the controversy over drugs, we will come to see it as a battle over unreal issues in which the real issues — the ones that matter to us as individuals — are completely skewed. Pro- and anti-drug forces are polarized in appearance, but in reality both are partly right and partly wrong. The more we start to talk about consciousness rather than about drugs, the more, I think, we will be able to see how much in agreement we are.

In these next chapters I will be talking about two very different ways of using the mind, but I will never be talking about two different groups of people. It seems to me that deep thinking, like daydreaming, is a natural component of consciousness that all of us have available to us all the time. Therefore, I am uninterested in questions like, Are you a deeper thinker than I am? or, Is she more capable of deep thinking than he is? The only question worth thinking about is, In the moment-to-moment situations of everyday life, do I use my mind in a deep way or in a straight way?

I will attempt to depict straight thinking, first by listing its characteristics, then by giving examples of conceptions that it has produced in our world. I will describe deep thinking in a similar way. At the outset I must emphasize that deep thinking predominates naturally in states of consciousness other than the ordinary, ego-centered waking state; consequently, it correlates with drug use only to the extent that drugs are used intelligently as tools to enter altered states of consciousness. I know a great many persons who use a great many drugs and yet think in straight ways most of the time. (In fact, excessive use of drugs is, itself, a pattern of behavior arising from straight conceptions.) On the other hand, I know a number of people who are very much at home in the lunar mind and yet have never used drugs; they make use of other methods of getting into altered states of consciousness. I know no people who are deep thinkers who do not spend significant portions of their mental life in nonordinary states of consciousness.

Straight thinking is ordinary thinking. It is what all of us do most of the time with our minds when we are normally alert and functioning in the world. It is what our conventional educational systems reward us for doing well. It is the kind of thinking that predominates in most of the institutions of our society at the present time. We are so used to it that many of us do not suspect the existence of another way of interpreting our perceptions of the world around us. In the same way, when the sun is high in the sky, the moon is invisible, and we have difficulty imagining moonlight.

I understand straight thinking for two reasons. First, like everyone I know, I engage in it frequently. Second, over the past few years, as I have more consciously explored other states of consciousness, I have become acutely aware of the straightness of much of the thinking in areas I am most familiar with: particularly science, medicine, and government. Wherever it appears, this kind of thinking has five identifiable characteristics, which I prefer to describe as "tendencies," since they vary in strength of expression but are always present in some degree.

1. A tendency to know things through the intellect rather than through some other faculty of the mind

People stuck in the solar mind tend to forget that the intellect is only one component of the mind; therefore, they think they know something completely when they understand it intellectually. The counterculture violently opposes this attitude and insists that direct experience is the only valid source of knowledge. In its more extreme forms, this insistence looks like simple anti-intellectualism and clearly frightens intellectuals. But in its more positive aspects, the countercultural emphasis on direct experience seems to me a breath of fresh air that is beginning to dispel some of the stagnation of intellectual life in our society. Indeed, those in academic communities who are open to new ways of thinking recognize its potential value to their own fields of inquiry. For example, Dr. Thomas R. Blackburn, a professor of chemistry, wrote in an article in *Science* in June 1971:

> ... the salient feature of the counterculture is its epistemology of direct sensuous experience, subjectivity, and respect for intuition — especially intuitive knowledge based on a "naïve" openness to nature and to other people. Both on its own merits and as a reaction to the abuses of technology, the movement has attracted increasing numbers of intelligent and creative students and professional people. I believe that science as a creative endeavor cannot survive the loss of these people; nor, without them, can science contribute to the solution of the staggering social and ecological problems that we face.
>   ... much of the criticism directed at the current scientific model of nature is quite valid. If society is to begin to enjoy the promise of the "scientific revolution," or even to survive in a tolerable form, science must change.[1]

Having identified with the role of intellectual for much of my life, I have found it difficult to accept the fact that my intellect may be a hindrance to the kind of development of my mind I now wish to undertake. But I now understand that the intellect is merely the thought producer of the mind and that thoughts are not realities. In order to perceive reality directly, one must sooner or later learn how to abandon the intellect and disengage oneself from the thoughts it produces incessantly. All instructional materials on meditation stress this theme. For example, in his manual, *Concentration and Meditation*, Christmas Humphreys warns the beginner:

> A more difficult problem, because entirely new, will be the claims of the intellect, which, with the antagonism displayed by every vehicle when it is sought for the first time to bring it under control, will fight for self-existence with an amazing variety of subtle wiles and unsound arguments. With an arrogance peculiar to itself it will strive to persuade the meditator that in this sphere alone lies truth, and it is all too noticeable that the West as a whole is a victim of this arrogance. Yet the intellect in itself is but a moulder of forms, and sooner or later consciousness must rise above the limitations which form implies . . . To such an extent are most of us dominated by the intellect, or "thought-machine," that in the early stages of meditation we fail to appreciate how it is deceiving us. Many a student imagines, for example, that he is meditating upon his chosen subject, only to find on strict analysis that the real object of his meditation is "I am meditating upon so and so!"[2]

Perhaps the most effective stratagem of the intellect is to convince its owner that it is equivalent to the mind; if one accepts this notion, abandoning the intellect becomes equivalent to losing one's mind. For this reason, intellectuals tend to look upon persons who have gone beyond the intellect as unfortunates who have suffered a mental catastrophe, even though those persons may have greater awareness than any intellectual can have.

Being able to abandon the intellect at will in order to experience

certain things directly does not mean losing the intellect perma-
nently. It is always there, always producing its endless chains of
associated thoughts, and always available for use. And thoughts
can be useful. After all, it was my intellect that led me to mescaline
by way of Huxley's *Doors of Perception* (although the motivation to
read up on the subject originated in a nonrational intuition that
mescaline was somehow important to me). But once the intellect
leads us to the brink of an experience, it has served its function,
and we must let go of it; otherwise, we never have the experience
and never come to know what we are talking about.

As a hallmark of straight thinking, attachment to the intellect is
especially visible in American academic communities. In my first
year at Harvard College I was a student in the Linguistics Department, under the chairmanship of the late Joshua Whatmough. In
one of the lectures I attended in his course, "Language," he ridiculed the idea that there could be such a thing as an "ineffable" experience. If an experience could not be expressed in words, he told
the class, it could not exist. He was very sure of himself and obviously unwilling to be contradicted. But a few weeks before, when I
had tried mescaline for the second time, I had had an experience
that certainly felt ineffable to me. There seemed to be no point in
trying to convey anything of its nature to Professor Whatmough;
instead I transferred out of the Linguistics Department into psychology, where people turned out to be even less interested in conscious experience. (They were strict behaviorists, experimenting
with rats and pigeons.) It should not be surprising that large numbers of young people, who are beginning to discover the advantages of direct experience, are becoming much less tolerant of the
conventional academic exercises of American colleges. As one's
thinking becomes less straight by virtue of conscious time spent
out of ordinary waking consciousness (regardless of the means
used to get out), one is no longer content with intellectual, verbal
descriptions of reality; direct experience becomes more and more
worth seeking. This is my own finding based on my own experi-

ence (if you will, on my personal research), and I cannot expect any reader to accept it as true until he can confirm it from his or her own experience. All I can do is present an intellectual argument explaining why it is true, which might lead the reader to design the appropriate experiments to test the proposition. To claim that my argument proved the proposition would be to fall into the same error of thinking made by so many university professors.

In any case, here is the argument: the essence of intellection is the generation of hypotheses about reality by a process of inductive reasoning — that is, by generalizing from observation. Only by direct experience can we confirm or reject these hypotheses with confidence. This kind of testing by actual trial is the strict meaning of the word *proof,* as one can detect in such uses as "proving grounds." In fact, the exception that proves the rule is not, as in the popular mind, the one that is always there and thus establishes proof automatically but rather the one that *tries* the worthiness of the hypothesis. If the conclusion about reality reached intellectually fails the test of confrontation with reality, then it must be rejected. Until the test is carried out, the hypothesis must be regarded as no more than a hypothesis. Some hypotheses are wrong — that is, divergent from reality. If a wrong hypothesis is used as the premise of subsequent intellectual activity or behavior, that activity and behavior will also be wrong, and the wrongness will increase the further one goes from the erroneous hypothesis. This significant risk of building wrong hypotheses into one's conceptual framework is the trouble with straight thinking. It arises directly from this first characteristic of straight thinking: identification of the mind with the intellect and acceptance of intellectual descriptions of reality as true without submitting them to the proof of trial by actual experiment. This false identification is itself an aspect of a more general false identification: the confusion of the mind with ordinary, ego-centered waking consciousness. In fact, all of the other characteristics of straight thinking

follow from this ultimate confusion because they are really characteristics of the ego and its thought-producing component, the intellect.*

2. A tendency to be attached to the senses and through them to external reality

Our senses bring us a great deal of information every moment
about the reality outside our heads. This sensory data is the primary source of information for ego consciousness and the intellect. In fact, the ego seems unable to disengage itself from the
moment-to-moment inflow of sensations arising from external reality. Consequently, it is only in states of consciousness other than
the ordinary waking state that we can have the experience of being
detached from these sensations. As I suggested earlier, detachment from external reality is a common characteristic of many altered states of consciousness. Most of us understand this correlation so well that we say a person is "somewhere else" when he is
daydreaming (that is, when he is in a light trance and is tuned out
of external reality), and we assure ourselves that a subject is in a
trance by waving a hand in front of his open eyes and getting no
response. Where is a person's consciousness when it is "some-

* These considerations explain to me a number of interesting reactions I have seen
people have to drugs. To the extent that an individual takes a drug to get himself out of
ego-centered consciousness (that is, to the extent that he is set to interpret the pharma-
cologic effects of the drug as an opportunity to experience some other sort of consciousness), to that extent will his ego rightly perceive the effects of the drug as threatening. Persons who are strongly attached to their egos, especially when trying drugs for
the first time or learning to use them, may defend themselves from this perceived
threat with a resurgence of intellectual activity. For example, when I first began smoking marijuana regularly with friends (in 1965–66), our highs, though enjoyable, were
extremely verbal. It was only after several years that I was able to learn to use marijuana
as an occasion for entering a meditative state in which I could ignore the verbal produc-
tions of my intellect. Similarly, I have seen individuals become compulsive talkers on
first exposure to hallucinogens, attain insight that this behavior represents resistance
to letting go, and on subsequent occasions learn to be quiet under the influence of the
drug. These observations are consistent with the supposition that attachment to intellect is a way of holding on to ego-centered consciousness and thus remaining straight.

where else"? If our conscious life is totally attached to our sensory perceptions of external reality, it is very likely that we will come to equate reality with external reality, just as we tend to equate mind with intellect, and consciousness with ordinary waking consciousness. The very existence of altered states of consciousness is a powerful piece of evidence that "proves" the rule equating reality with external reality and finds it wanting.

The experience of people who learn to retain conscious memories of trances, dreams, highs, and meditations is that another kind of reality exists, perhaps with many variations, that we can call internal or nonordinary reality, or lunar mind. It is precisely that aspect of reality we are unconscious of when in the ordinary waking state, and the unconscious mind is precisely that part of the mind that pays attention to it.

In the contact I have had with academic psychiatry in several "good" institutions in Boston and San Francisco, I have been struck by the fact that many psychiatrists, even though they talk constantly of the unconscious mind and are always speculating on the unconscious thoughts of their patients, appear to know this part of the mind only as an intellectual construct and not through direct experience. Furthermore, many of them appear to be both fascinated with and frightened by people who have open access to their unconscious minds, particularly if they have gained this access by using drugs. This anxiety among psychiatrists is a significant problem in the profession as it is now constituted and is clearly the source of the irrationality that pervades much psychiatric thinking about drugs and altered states of consciousness — the kind of irrationality we examined previously in considering arguments made by psychiatrists against the use of drugs.

It is also clear that this kind of fear is not restricted to any profession. Any mind functioning in a straight way feels threatened by the implications of states of consciousness that point to the existence of another kind of reality. The ego rightly senses the threat implied to its dominion by the fact of an unconscious mind that can perceive an internal reality. Yet nonordinary reality can be experienced even though it cannot be understood intellectually. And this concept of a reality that is beyond human knowledge but nevertheless can be experienced directly seems to me to be the precise sense of the word *mystery* as it used to describe rites like the Eleusinian mysteries of ancient Greece.

We have an excellent example of the incomprehensibility of nonordinary reality from the point of view of ego consciousness in the popular book *The Teachings of Don Juan* by Carlos Castaneda. In 1965 Castaneda apprenticed himself to a Yaqui Indian witch doctor (*brujo*) from central Mexico who initiated him into mysteries associated with several magic plants. Among the plants was devil's weed (*Datura meteloides*), a relative of henbane and deadly nightshade, all of which contain similar alkaloids and all of which were used in medieval witchcraft ceremonies to trigger unusual states of consciousness. A common experience of participants in these ceremonies was that of flying through the air. Under don Juan's direction, and like the witches of old, Castaneda anointed his body with an extract of devil's weed mixed with fat. He described his subsequent experience as follows:

> Don Juan kept staring at me. I took a step toward him. My legs were rubbery and long, extremely long. I took another step. My knee joints felt springy, like a vault pole; they shook and vibrated and contracted elastically. I moved forward. The motion of my body was slow and shaky; it was more like a tremor forward and up. I looked down and saw don Juan sitting below me, way below me. The momentum carried me forward one more step, which was even more elastic and longer than the preceding one. And from there I soared. I remember coming down once; then I pushed up with both feet, sprang backward, and glided on my back. I saw the dark sky above me and the clouds going by me. I jerked my body so I could look down. I saw the dark mass of the mountains. My speed was extraordinary. My arms were fixed, folded against my sides. My head was the directional unit. If I kept it bent backward I made vertical circles. I changed directions by turning my head to the side. I enjoyed such freedom and swiftness as I had never known before.

The experience ended with Castaneda coming down to earth, becoming sick, and losing awareness. The next day he had the following conversation with his mentor:

... I had to ask him, "Did I really fly, don Juan?"

"That is what you told me. Didn't you?"

"I know, don Juan. I mean, did my body fly? Did I take off like a bird?"

"You always ask me questions I cannot answer. You flew. That is what the second portion of the devil's weed is for. As you take more of it, you will learn to fly perfectly. It is not a simple matter. A man *flies* with the help of the second portion of the devil's weed. That is all I can tell you. What you want to know makes no sense. Birds fly like birds and a man who has taken the devil's weed flies as such."

"As birds do?"

"No, he flies as a man who has taken the weed."

"Then I didn't really fly, don Juan. I flew in my mind alone. Where was my body?"

"In the bushes," he replied cuttingly, but immediately broke into laughter again. "The trouble with you is that you understand things in only one way. You don't think a man flies; and yet a brujo can move a thousand miles in one second to see what is going on. He can deliver a blow to his enemies long distances away. So, does he or doesn't he fly?"

"You see, don Juan, you and I are differently oriented. Suppose, for the sake of argument, one of my fellow students had been here with me when I took the devil's weed. Would he have been able to see me flying?"

"There you go again with your questions about what would happen if . . . It is useless to talk that way. If your friend, or anybody else, takes the second portion of the weed all he can do is fly. Now, if he had simply watched you, he might have seen you flying, or he might not. That depends on the man."

"But what I mean, don Juan, is that if you and I look at a bird and see it fly, we agree that it is flying. But if two of my friends had seen me flying as I did last night, would they have agreed that I was flying?"

"Well, they might have. You agree that birds fly because you have seen them flying. Flying is a common thing with birds. But you will not agree on many other things birds do, because you have never seen birds doing them. If your friends knew about men flying with the devil's weed, then they would agree."

"Let's put it another way, don Juan. What I meant to say is that if I had tied myself to a rock with a heavy chain I would have flown just the same, because my body had nothing to do with my flying."

Don Juan looked at me incredulously. "If you tie yourself to a rock," he said, "I'm afraid you will have to fly holding the rock with its heavy chain."[3]

Castaneda never seems to get the point that his experience of nonordinary reality is no less real for being unverifiable in the realm of ordinary experience. Internal reality, in all of its varied forms, is a different order of reality that is self-validating. And the most elementary requirement for getting in touch with it is simple withdrawal of attention from sensory attachment to external reality.

It should not be surprising to learn, therefore, that such withdrawal is emphasized in all instructional materials on meditation. In fact, Patanjali in his ancient codification of yoga listed sense withdrawal *(Pratyahara)* as one of the basic eight "limbs" of the system. A modern commentator on his aphorisms writes:

> Pratyahara is a detaching of the mind from the sense-organs. The word means "gathering towards." It checks the outgoing powers of the mind and turns them inwards. It is a gathering in and integration of the previously scattered mental energies. In Pratyahara one frees oneself from the thraldom of the sense-organs.[4]

The experience of sense withdrawal is one we have all had if we have ever fallen into a reverie in a room with a ticking clock. The clock continues to tick, the ear continues to hear it, but the mind ceases to pay attention. Masters of meditation assure us that with practice we can learn to detach our minds at will from all of our senses. The worth of this accomplishment is stated tersely in the *Bhagavad-Gita,* in which Krishna (the Hindu analog of Jesus) says:

"The tortoise can draw in his legs:/ The seer can draw in his senses. I call him illumined."[5]

As a final comment on the matter of sensory attachment as a defining characteristic of straight thinking, I would note that drug experiences, particularly with marijuana and psychedelics, may be more or less determined by sensations arising from external reality and that there is no question in my mind that sensory or "esthetic" experiences with drugs are less profound than other kinds. Just as a surge of intellectual activity may serve as a defensive maneuver of the ego to strengthen its control of experience when that control is threatened, so may absorption in sensory phenomena serve the same function. Psychiatrists who have used drugs like LSD and psilocybin in psychotherapy stress the importance of guiding patients beyond the realm of esthetic experience into the deeper and more interesting realms of the psyche.

3. A tendency to pay attention to outward forms rather than to inner contents and thus to lapse into materialism

Attachment to senses, as we have seen, leads to acceptance of the hypothesis that external reality constitutes all of reality. Concomitant with the acceptance of this false premise is the belief that something has been experienced or known when its outward appearance has registered on the mind through the senses. It is this ultimate confusion of appearance with reality that necessarily leads to materialistic formulations of human life and the cosmos. By *materialism* I do not mean a passion for acquiring fast cars and home theaters, although the acquisitive lust of modern Americans may well be a symptom of what I have in mind. Rather, I mean the tendency to see material reality as more important or more basic than nonmaterial reality — a tendency I have pointed out in previous chapters in connection with the notions of pharmacologists about the relationship between events in the physical body and brain and conscious experiences.

The essence of materialism is the attribution of causality to external, physical reality. In this way, psychosis becomes a matter of disordered biochemistry or brain function; a high is due to the presence of a drug in the body; infectious disease is caused by germs, and so on. The problem with formulations of this kind is simply that they fail to give us the power to describe, predict, and control the phenomena of external reality, as we saw again and again in our earlier analyses of conventional theories of drugs. Incorrect attribution of causality — so easy to spot in pharmacological descriptions of drug effects once one knows to look for it — is nothing more than a specific instance of the more general error of thinking I have described as the equation of reality with external, material reality.

Since this false equation is, itself, a consequence of the equation of consciousness with ego, it should be clear how the initial divergence from reality of a general premise grows with subsequent reasoning based upon that premise. Materialistic conceptions are so divergent from reality that they leave us unable to modify the world around us except for the worse. (I will give specific examples in a few moments.) Still, they are not the end of the chain of false reasoning I have called straight thinking; the compounding of errors goes on to its logical conclusion.

4. A tendency to perceive differences rather than similarities between phenomena

A root function of the intellect is discrimination and classification — a function based upon the perception of differences in the appearances of things. This kind of intellectual activity has been very prominent in Western science, particularly in its analysis of the natural history of the world around us. Of course, there are times when it is useful to distinguish a mushroom from a toadstool or a white oak from a black oak. But the intellect, by itself, cannot stop this sort of activity, with the result that persons attached to intellect cannot stop perceiving differences. By contrast, persons who forsake ego consciousness, even for a moment, often have an overwhelming sense of the essential similarity of all things; indeed, this direct perception of unity is the very heart of mystic experience. It is not that the apparent differences disappear, rather, the mind experiences a sort of figure-ground reversal in which what had previously been sensed unconsciously as background becomes the central fact of perception. All people who have this experience directly (not those who understand it intellectually) testify that it is accompanied by powerful feelings of joy.

The ultimate distinction made by the intellect is that between *self* and *not-self*; the sense of I as distinct from everything else in the universe is the very root of ego consciousness. Furthermore, in the ego's own terms, all that is not-self is potentially threatening because it has the capacity to undermine the whole conceptual scheme built up so carefully by the intellect. Consequently, people who have not yet learned to let go of ego consciousness must necessarily experience the profound sense of isolation that some philosophers consider the normal human condition. Along with this existential loneliness comes the inevitable conviction that one is surrounded by a hostile universe. Everything out there that is not-self seems bent on destroying the fragile, isolated bubble of self. The joy that invariably accompanies mystic experience (or any other kind of ego loss) is simply the natural emotion that wells up when this sense of fearful isolation ends.

These thoughts are not merely theological abstractions. Let me illustrate them with an example from my own experience. Like many of my friends, I projected my sense of the hostility of nature onto certain insects, and while my fear of them did not approach phobic proportions, it was sufficient to keep me from relaxing completely in a wild setting. Although I did not understand it at the time, these feelings arose entirely from my conceiving of these insects (particularly bees and wasps) as fundamentally different from myself and, "therefore," able to harm me. Once, during an LSD trip, I found myself high and unattached to my ego in a field with many bees. For the first time in my life I experienced these creatures as essentially similar to myself and was able to see in them extraordinary beauty I had never before noticed. In the years since, I have learned to extend that feeling to most other insects. Especially interesting is my finding that the insects themselves appear to behave differently toward me. I now live in a country house around which hundreds of wasps and bees build their nests, and although I have frequent contact with them, even removing their nests when necessary from locations with heavy human traffic, I have never been stung and appear to cause them no discomfort or alarm. Needless to say, this change (which had its origin in an altered state of consciousness triggered by a drug) has been a source of great joy.

It is probably not necessary for me to point out that the tendency of the ego to focus on the differences rather than the similarities between itself and things out there can cause far worse troubles than differences with insects. The unsatisfactoriness of many human relationships and all acts of inhumanity are traceable directly to the same root problem. In fact, the mental step required before a human being commits violence against another human being appears to be definition of the other person as "other" or "different." This process seems all too natural when our minds are functioning in a straight way.

5. A tendency to negative thinking, pessimism, and despair

Undiluted straight thinking leads inevitably to despair. When you are living alone in a hostile universe, unable to change anything except for the worse, you can only lapse into increasingly negative and impotent states. Materialism represents a misunderstanding of cause and effect that automatically condemns the straight thinker to imprisonment in a darkening reality, and it is all too clear that this is precisely the experience of many contemporary Americans. Many of us can see nothing but imminent disaster in whatever direction we look — whether at the economy, at politics, at conditions in cities, at our own bodies, and, especially, at our own minds. And it is terribly difficult for the solar mind to comprehend that negative thinking is self-confirming. The more one is set to interpret perceptions negatively, the more evidence one finds that disaster is imminent; the more evidence one finds, the stronger one's conviction grows that this way of looking at things is right. Specifically because the ego cannot see the reality of nonordinary reality, straight thinkers cannot find the true causes of the negative manifestations of their own ways of perceiving. For the truth is that external phenomena are caused not by things out there (even though it looks that way to the ego) but rather by things in here — that is, in the unconscious, lunar mind, from which we are cut off whenever we think straight. All of the nightmares that contemporary ego consciousness can dream up — the nuclear holocausts, ecological disasters, race wars, global epidemics, and psychiatric catastrophes — will continue to come closer and closer to actual manifestation as long as the mental patterns that create them continue.

And this is, at last, the end of the chain of false logic that is straight thinking. Identification of consciousness with ego consciousness leads to confusion of mind with intellect, to acceptance of appearance as reality, to materialistic formulations of the interaction of mind and matter, to isolation and fear, to increasingly negative conceptions of reality, and, ultimately and very logically, to disaster. I do not know the etymology of the word *straight* in this context, but it seems to me a singularly appropriate adjective. Straight thinking is straight in the way an interstate highway is straight: unlike a winding country road it does not follow the natural contours of reality. And in its ever-widening divergence from reality it leads straight to impotence, despair, and death.

At this point I must hasten to add a note of reassurance. I have been talking about straight *thinking*, not straight thinkers. I am not condemning all of us to hell. All of us are straight thinkers some of the time, but all of us are deep thinkers, too. What I have just described are characteristics and consequences of pure straight thinking, unmodified by interaction with our unconscious life. The fact is that all of us spend time in nonordinary states of consciousness whether we use drugs or not; the trouble is, simply, that most of us have been discouraged from maintaining continuous awareness of these states. Thus we tend to compartmentalize and isolate those very factors that can temper ego consciousness and get us out of the straight bind. Many of us get locked into ordinary consciousness, but we all have the key to freedom.

It is one thing to characterize straight thinking, another to see it at work in everyday life. Here follow actual examples of conceptions produced by straight logic that all of us might subscribe to.

1. The use of insecticides to control insects

In describing my experiences with insects, I emphasized that the process was purely internal: I changed my fears of insects and the nature of their interaction with me by doing certain operations inside my head — in particular, by experiencing the insects I was afraid of through a state of consciousness other than my usual ego-centered one. An alternative was available to me, of course, one that I had made frequent use of in the past. I could have picked up an aerosol can of insecticide and killed the insects that came near me. I now find the alternative unacceptable, and I make that judgment without recourse to any consideration of the morality or immorality of killing insects.

Insecticides, as chemicals poisonous to living organisms, are more meaningful to me as concrete symbols of straight thinking than they are as mere physical substances to have around the house or garden. For they are the manifestations of a way of thinking that imagines hostile appearances of nature can be banished by direct applications of force. And, significantly, it is deadly force that is brought to bear. But, as any cell physiologist can testify, the ways in which our own cellular life processes differ from those of insects are much less important than the ways in which they are similar. Consequently, the application of cellular poisons to our houses and food must, in a very real way, be hurting ourselves, regardless of the amount of damage we can now measure. It cannot be good; the only question is, How bad is it? So the first strike against this way of dealing with insects is that it directly rebounds on us.

Moreover, does the method even achieve the desired objective? The goal is not really to get rid of particular individuals of the insect order but rather to make a negative manifestation of nature go away. Now, as vigorous selective agents, insecticides in our world are playing a significant role in the evolutionary development of all insect species. They neatly weed out susceptible members, concentrating in insect gene pools all over the world the genetic factors conferring resistance to these chemicals. Thus the use of insecticides, by straightforward principles of natural selection, creates new races of insects, resistant to these substances and often more aggressive or tough in other ways. Already, we have gotten into fast-moving arms races with a number of species in which resistance has escalated to match escalations of toxicity. In some cases, the patterns of insect destruction of crops are now more devastating than before powerful insecticides were first used years ago. The method looks as if it works in the short run because it seems to dispose of all the visible pests immediately. But the long-range evaluation is unnerving. Not only does the method not make the hostile manifestation disappear; it directly makes it take worse forms.

Here we are at the last stop on the chain of false logic. The idea that we can make things we do not like go away by forcing them out of existence leads to action that harms us directly while making the things even less likable. Seen in retrospect, my way of solving the same problem was to accept insects as they were, to locate in my mind the source of negative interpretation of my perceptions of them, and then to disaffiliate my mind from that source (which meant the dissociation of consciousness from ego). As soon as I did that, insects were no longer the same. And they have been getting less the same ever since. In fact, they are turning into positive manifestations of nature. Meanwhile, the believer in insecticides must go on fighting a never-ending battle, his way of thinking leading him ever onward to frustration and despair.

2. The use of antibiotics

The parallel between antibiotics and insecticides is so striking that it requires little comment. In their importance as selective agents modifying the evolution of bacteria, antibiotics are strictly analogous to chemical poisons used to control insects. Their increasing use over the past thirty years correlates exactly with the appearance of greater and greater numbers of organisms that are more virulent in their parasitic relationships with man and terribly adept at developing resistance to the latest antibiotics from the world's pharmaceutical laboratories. Hospital infections with these virulent strains have been rising sharply, as all medical personnel know. In my years of hospital work I saw many deaths of debilitated patients following recurrent hospital-borne infections, each bout following the application of the stronger antibiotic given to hold the last bout in check.

Predictably, the more powerful antibiotics are much more toxic to human cells and can be as dangerous to life as a generalized infection. Penicillin, the first true antibiotic to be discovered, interferes with the cell-wall formation of certain bacteria, and bacterial cell walls (the *outer surfaces* of the cell) are different in important ways from human cell walls. But many newer, more powerful antibiotics are toxic to basic cellular processes — processes we have in common with bacteria. Here again, the action suggested by straight thinking injures us directly and worsens the problem it was meant to solve.

But is there an alternative to killing bacteria? The analog of the process I used on insects may not suggest itself immediately. Yet it is available and is just as effective. To explain it, I must first point out the straightness of allopathy.

3. Allopathic medicine

Allopathy is the system of medicine I was taught at Harvard. It is the system of medicine medical doctors are taught the world over. And few allopaths ever stop to consider that their system is not the only possible one.

The unifying principle of allopathic practice is its philosophy of treating illness by counteracting the symptoms of illness. Thus if high blood pressure is a manifestation of disease, antihypertensive drugs are administered; if serious inflammation occurs on the surface of the body, antiinflammatory medications are applied. And so on and so on: this is the essence of the allopathic method. Now, "counteracting the symptoms of illness" has a very straight sound to it. *Counteract* suggests the use of force to make negative manifestations disappear, and *symptoms* suggests superficial appearance rather than inner reality. And, indeed, the supposition that our dominant system of medicine is based in straight thinking is easy to confirm.

What I am about to say I write as a man trained fully in general allopathic medicine. I undertook this training as a continuation of what I saw as my general education, not as a step toward entering a particular profession. For the past two years I have been dissociated completely from the world of allopathic practice, during which time I have thought much about my experiences in it. My retrospective impression of allopathy is that it is unable to control well the phenomena of health and illness and that it often unwittingly intensifies manifestations of illness rather than ameliorates them. Such has been my own experience over the course of five years. I do not expect readers who are allopathic practitioners or patients to accept my view on faith any more than I expect law-enforcement agents or committed drug users to accept without proof my earlier views about the dangers of drugs. But I do ask all readers to give these arguments thought and to test them against their own experience. I must also say that I have met many intelligent, sensitive allopathic physicians who are genuinely dedicated to alleviating human suffering (some of whom unconsciously use nonallopathic methods to produce real cures). Furthermore, in rejecting allopathy as a theoretical system, I do not claim to have all the answers. There is much about health and illness I still do not understand, much knowledge I am still seeking. But I feel confident in making certain criticisms of the approach to disease that now predominates in our medical schools and hospitals.

Modern allopathic medicine is essentially materialistic. For example, the widely accepted germ theory of disease — a cornerstone of allopathic theory — states that certain microscopic entities (bacteria and viruses are the most important) whose appearance in space and time correlates well with other physical manifestations of illness are causative of illness. Therefore, the theory continues, infectious illness can profitably be treated by trying to force these entities out of existence. One of the great contributors to this theory was the German bacteriologist and Nobel laureate Robert Koch (1843–1910), author of a masterpiece of straight logic known to all allopaths as "Koch's Postulates." Medical students are required to accept these dogmas on faith, to recite them faithfully on examinations, and to interpret their observations of infectious disease through them. Here they are, as presented in the text I used in my microbiology course at Harvard:

> How can one prove that a given microorganism really causes a disease? Traditionally, the etiologic [i.e., causative] relationship between a microorganism and a disease is established by fulfilling "Koch's Postulates": (1) The microorganism must regularly be isolated from cases of the illness. (2) It must be grown in pure culture *in vitro* [i.e., in a test tube]. (3) When such a pure culture is inoculated into susceptible animal species, the typical disease must result. (4) From such experimentally induced disease the microorganism must again be isolated.[6]

Actually, fulfillment of these postulates does no more than establish correlation between the presence of the germ in the body and the other physical manifestations of the illness as observed in animals. It does not prove that real-world patients get the same physical illness because they come into contact with the germ. You may ask, Doesn't fulfillment of Postulate Three prove cause? The animal was healthy before the germ was put into it and sick afterward. True. But inoculation of germs into animals (usually by injection) is an unnatural procedure that obscures the relevance of any subsequent observations to the world beyond the laboratory.

In our consideration of research on drugs, we saw that experimental rigor obtained at the expense of relevance to the world at large is of questionable value because it increases the risk of formulating hypotheses that explain the data but are of no real use to us. We live in a world full of germs, some of which are correlated with physical symptoms of infectious disease. But only some of us get infectious diseases some of the time. Why? Because there are factors in *us* that determine what kind of a relationship we will have with those germs that are always out there — a relationship of balanced coexistence or one of unbalanced antagonism. Furthermore, outside of laboratories scientists do not (usually) go around inoculating us with potentially dangerous microorganisms. Fulfillment of the third of Koch's Postulates bypasses the whole system by which relationships with germs are internally determined. I admit that it looks as if germs cause disease, but remember: acceptance of appearance for reality is a distinguishing feature of straight thinking. It also looks as if drugs cause highs, and people who accept that proposition get into trouble.

My experiences in allopathic medicine, both as a patient and as a practitioner, have led me to conclude that all illness is psychosomatic. I do not use the word in the sense of "unreal" or "phony," as many allopaths do. Rather, I mean that all illness has both psychic and physical components, and it seems to me that the physical manifestations of illness (including the appearance of germs in tissues) are always effects, while the causes always lie within the realm of the mind, albeit the unconscious mind. In other words, the disease process seems to me to be initiated often by changes in

consciousness. In the case of infectious illness, the initial causative change is not that germs come to attack the body but that
something happens in the person that permits a breakdown of the
normal harmonious balance between the body and the microorganisms surrounding it.

For example, the staphylococci that seem to cause boils are normal inhabitants of our skins. Most of the time, their relationship
to us is symbiotic — mutually beneficial. Occasionally, that balance breaks down and boils appear. The problem is to restore the
balance, not to make the staph germs disappear. An allopath,
thinking that the germs cause the boils, treats this condition by
trying to make the germs go away, by giving antibiotics. But antibiotics merely kill off the germs that are most inclined to form harmonious relationships with us, leaving behind the more aggressive, tougher ones that are less inclined to enter into balanced
existence with their hosts. Allopathic hospitals are virtual factories
for turning out new strains of staph that are not only highly resistant to several generations of antibiotics but also much more ruth-
less in their attacks on human beings.

Here is a familiar pattern. In attempting to control insects and
germs by reliance on external, material substances, we meet with
initial success and eventual failure. Sooner or later the substances
fail us, and we find ourselves in a worse state than before. Many
times, our use of materials becomes more and more desperate
when we see them begin not to work and do not understand why
they are not working. In our desperation, we often look for better
or stronger substances. I can see no essential difference between
this pattern and that of drug dependence. The user who depends
on drugs to get into desirable states of consciousness becomes tolerant to them and cannot maintain his highs. If he fails to realize
the nature of his problem, his use of drugs becomes more and
more desperate, and he must search for something stronger. In
other words, drug dependence — far from being an isolated phenomenon caused by particular substances — is simply a special
case of a very general problem: reliance on external things to pro-

duce or maintain desired internal states (including highs, health, and freedom from anxiety about manifestations of nature). The name of this problem is materialism; its consequence is always the same; its cause is straight thinking.

In suggesting that infectious illness is actually initiated by psychic changes, I am not invoking mystical forces. Consciousness, as I have said repeatedly, is real, and it has connections to every part of the body by way of the peripheral nerves. An unconscious impulse can easily be transmitted through the nervous system to the skin (or any other tissue), where it can cause changes resulting in the breakdown of equilibrium between us and the microorganisms we encounter. Conversely, equilibrium can be restored by transmitting other impulses along the same pathways, and this principle is the basis of nonallopathic healing, of which I shall have more to say in the next chapter. Unfortunately for allopaths, this kind of true healing (I have now seen a number of impressive cases) involves the transmission of consciousness through a branch of the nervous system — the autonomic nervous system — that allopathic medicine regards as "involuntary," that is, beyond the reach of consciousness. Thus, allopaths are prisoners of their own conceptions of the mind and body and will never discover this other sort of healing until they give up those conceptions. In medicine as elsewhere, straight thinking leads to an inability to describe, predict, or control external reality accurately and to an inability to see the reality of the direction in which the solution lies.

That there is a great deal wrong with the medical system of this country is no secret. We see all around us the manifestations of this wrongness: the impossible economics of the system, its inability to deliver medical care to those who need it most, the unwieldiness of its educational curriculums, and, most of all, its inability to make us a healthy society. The incidence of major killing diseases — heart disease, cancer, and stroke — continues to climb; the illnesses directly caused by allopathic methods and hospital practices get worse and worse; and the newest techniques of the system — I would single out organ transplants as a prime example — seem to be going in directions that are less and less natural. And because allopaths have no grip on the true causes of disease they cannot prevent us from getting sick; they can only treat our acute problems. I know a number of young physicians who see themselves as founders of a revolution in American medicine. They are very vocal about the curriculums of medical schools, the lack of good medical care, overcrowded hospitals, the rigidity of the profession, and so forth. But they fail to see that these symptoms of ill health of the system are but the superficial manifestations of something very wrong at the core. And as these young doctors fight to counteract those symptoms, they go on parroting and believing materialistic nonsense like Koch's Postulates, which are much more representative of the core problem. The real revolution in medicine, like all real revolutions, will go on at the level of conceptions.

4. The allopathic model in psychiatry

I have already mentioned that I consider much of conventional psychiatry straight. Perhaps the best indication of its straightness has been its ready acceptance of the allopathic medical model in its approach to disturbances of the mind. Psychiatry today is a branch of allopathic medicine because psychiatrists themselves choose to be in that position. In the early years of this century psychiatrists imagined that affiliation with allopaths would make them more legitimate in the eyes of the public, and so they decided to require medical training of students seeking entrance to their professional academies. This strategy has made the profession a success but has led most psychiatrists to think of mental disturbances in straight terms.

For example, certain mental processes, like neuroses, which are normal phases of psychic development with strongly positive potential, are regarded negatively as manifestations of illness to be made to go away. Now, the essence of neurosis is ambivalence — the simultaneous experience of opposite feelings. Ego consciousness cannot make sense of ambivalence because the ego, in its self/not-self classifications, thinks in terms of either/or. Consequently, ambivalence (a very real feeling) is threatening to the ego because it violates straight logic. The problem, then, is not the ambivalence but the way one looks at it. And if one looks at it only from the point of view of ego-centered waking consciousness, it looks so frightening that one can easily lapse into kinds of inaction and depression that seem to confirm the supposition that one is sick. All too often, this view is reinforced in treatment with conventional psychiatrists, many of whom see their function as strengthening the egos of their patients to resist neurotic conflicts. Like their medical counterparts, these allopathic psychiatrists use techniques that can make patients worse rather than better — the usual inverted consequence of action based on straight conceptions. In the next chapter I will suggest a very different way of conceiving of neurosis, one based on different premises and a positive viewpoint.

5. Political action as a means of producing external change

The use of political force, whether by those in power or those out of power, to effect changes in societies seems to me to be unmistakably analogous to all of the other variants of the straight model we have considered. And like them, it seems only to rebound on its users and make worse the very manifestations it is intended to improve. Americans have had an excellent chance to grasp this principle over the past few years, but to see it requires emotional detachment from *both* sides. As soon as one achieves this detachment, it is instantly clear that government repression directly increases the phenomena it is meant to suppress while antigovernment activity directly brings on further repression — an escalating cycle strictly parallel to those we have seen with insects and insecticides, bacteria and antibiotics. It is an invariable consequence of trying to effect changes in the world working from assumptions that are divergent from reality.

I hope the straightness of these examples is clear. In every case it arises from the confusion of our perceptions of reality with reality itself, from the formulation of erroneous hypotheses that do not conform to our own direct experience. I hope also that these examples convey something of the power of straight thinking in our world; at the moment it is the rule, not the exception. I have several other examples to present, but all of them concern the central topic of this book — the drug problem — and I shall save them for later. Let us be done with straight thinking for now; there is a bright alternative to consider.

7. A Trip to the Moon: Deep Thinking

D EEP THINKING IS the mirror image of straight thinking. When we step into nonordinary reality even for a moment, we experience things directly, see inner contents rather than external forms, and suddenly find ourselves able to participate in changing reality for the better. This other way of interpreting perceptions comes first as episodic flashes, unpredictable, discontinuous. But the more flashes of it one has, the easier it becomes to maintain. And deep thinking is not something foreign that needs to be learned; it develops spontaneously as we unlearn habitual ways of using the mind.

It would be absurd to attempt to describe a way of thinking based in experience rather than description. Therefore, I will keep my comments about deep thinking to a minimum and instead will give a number of examples of conceptions it has led me to over the past few years. As briefly as possible, here are the essential components of the process:

1. Reliance on intuition as well as intellection

Intuition is something known to all of us by experience; to the intellect it is a mystery. In fact, intellectual speculation about the nature of intuition is in the same muddle it was when it started many years ago. Contemporary educational theorists recognize that intuition is the most important intrinsic factor governing acquisition of information in the growing child, but I am not impressed that they have developed effective methods of fostering this capacity in the process of education.

Intuitive flashes are transient, spontaneous altered states of consciousness consisting of particular sensory experiences or thoughts coupled with strong emotional reactions. But — and this is the distinguishing feature — the intellect cannot explain the association; there is no logical reason for the feelings we get on encountering certain persons, places, things, or ideas. Such real experiences, arising from the lunar mind, challenge the logic of ordinary, solar consciousness. So, in our ordinary waking state, we are uneasy about intuitive knowledge and, consequently, unable to describe it well, predict it well, or control it well.

If our ordinary conscious mind has no record of associations between certain experiences and certain feelings, where do these associations originate? They originate in the unconscious mind, and the strangeness of intuitions is the same strange feeling we experience whenever a portion of our unconscious life breaks through to our waking awareness. This sense of the nonordinary is strongest when it accompanies the purest forms of intuitions: unaccountable yet powerful convictions of knowing how things really are — of sensing directly that something is true. Probably, all people have such intuitions from time to time, but only some people act on them or bother to check on their usefulness. That is to say, only some of us trust our intuitions.

Now, the history of science makes clear that the greatest advancements in human understanding of the universe are made by intuitive leaps at the frontiers of knowledge, not by intellectual walks along well-traveled paths. Similarly, the greatest scientific thinkers are those who rely on sudden intuitive flashes to solve problems. Nevertheless, all of our universities attempt to train scientists by methods appropriate to the development of the intellect rather than the intuitive faculty.

In considering straight thinking, I noted that the essence of intellection is inductive reasoning: that is, the elaboration of general hypotheses from specific data provided by the senses. I suggested also that the problem with total reliance on this process is the danger of formulating hypotheses divergent from reality, failing to prove them by actual experiment, and using them as premises for subsequent reasoning and action. Teaching in science today relies exclusively on inductive procedures. For example, the entire preclinical curriculum of medical school is a mass of specific facts, observations, and experimental data, from which students of allopathy are expected to draw general conclusions regarding health and illness.

The looking-glass version of this process is deduction — that is, reasoning away from general premises to the specific case at hand. If the premises are known to be sound, the conclusions will be sound, too. And our intuitive faculty is nothing other than a source of sound premises about the nature of reality.

Learning to think deeply (or unlearning straight thinking) does not mean rejecting the intellect (a mistake made by some persons who wake up to the nature of straight thinking, then devote all of their energies to fighting it rather than developing a positive alternative). As a machine for producing thoughts, the intellect has a useful function if it is put in its proper place. And that place is coordinate with the intuitive faculty. As we become aware of our intuitions, learn to trust them, and then feed them into our intellects as premises, we begin to come up with very interesting and very useful ideas to guide us — useful because they lead us toward reality rather than away from it. This leads to unity in consciousness: the conjunction of solar mind and lunar mind.

This guiding function of intuition has been venerated by wise men throughout history. They have told us again and again, in legends and myths,* aphorisms, poems, and allegories, that there exists within us a source of direct information about reality that can teach us all we need to know. (Which is, after all, the literal meaning of the word *intuition*.) Maimonides called this source "the still, small voice." A Chinese sage, Hsuan-chiao, said of it: "You remain

* For a superb example with excellent commentary see the old Irish myth of Conn-Eda, "A Pagan Hero," in Heinrich Zimmer's *The King and the Corpse*, 2nd ed. (Joseph Campbell, ed., Bollingen Series XI, Princeton, New Jersey: Princeton University Press, 1956), pp. 26–52.

silent and it speaks,/You speak and it is silent." Many commentators call it superconsciousness to distinguish it from the "lower" (or subconscious) functions of the unconscious mind, such as the operation of the autonomic nervous system. And all of them stress that the only requirement for getting in touch with this source is the suspension of ordinary mental activity. We cannot make intuitions happen; we can only let them enter our awareness. In fact, if we disengage our awareness from ego consciousness and intellect, we cannot stop intuitive knowledge from bubbling up out of the unconscious depths. In daydreams, trances, reveries, meditations, we are much more open to our unconscious mind and to the inner teachings that come through it. And this openness obtains regardless of the means used to enter the altered states of consciousness. It is important to understand that the drug subculture in America, despite much superficial antiintellectualism, has provided many people with social support for becoming aware of and trusting their own intuitions — something the dominant culture has failed to do. Coordination of intellection with intuition, with increased reliance on deductive reasoning, is the outstanding characteristic of deep thinking. The other characteristics I will now mention follow from this first because they are really based on specific intuitions that come to us when we leave ordinary consciousness behind.

2. Acceptance of the ambivalent nature of things

Ambivalence is the coexistence of opposites that appear to be mutually antagonistic. Straight thinking with its either/or logic cannot understand this phenomenon, much less accept it and derive benefit from it. But as soon as we tune out our intellects and connect with our intuitive sources of knowledge, we discover that ambivalence is part of the way things are. In commenting on the "universal law of co-existing opposites," Heinrich Zimmer, an Asian scholar, has written: ". . . completeness consists in opposites co-operating through conflict . . . the pattern of existence is woven of antagonistic co-operation, alternations of ascendancy and decline . . . it is built of bright *and* dark, day *and* night — *Yang* and *Yin*, in the Chinese formulation."[1]

The idea that reality manifests itself to us in the guise of pairs of opposites is a very old one. It appears frequently in Eastern philosophies and religions, and in the Western tradition is traceable back to the Garden of Eden, where it takes the form of the Tree of Knowledge of Good and Evil. Modern physicists have pursued this paradoxical dualism into the subatomic world, where they find that entities like electrons and photons can exist either as waves or particles, energy or matter.

The problem is not that things have this ambivalent nature, but that our ordinary consciousness cannot accept it. Lunar consciousness, however, is perfectly capable of substituting a both/ and formulation for the either/or of the ego. In fact, in altered states of consciousness people often experience pairs of opposites simultaneously and find the experience very worthwhile.

Here is a mundane example: some years ago I took a dose of LSD in Death Valley on a night of the full moon in July. One of my most vivid recollections of the night is that I could not tell whether I was warm or cold because I had both sensations simultaneously and powerfully. Furthermore, this simultaneous experience of opposite sensations was intimately bound up with a state of egolessness and timelessness, and a tremendously increased ability to concentrate. I do not believe these effects were pharmacological; I have experienced them since that time without having taken any drug, most memorably on coming out of a very intense sweat lodge on the Rosebud (Lakota) Reservation in South Dakota one frigid November day. I had exactly the same feelings, including the experience of being simultaneously warm and cold.

The point is that when we enter nonordinary reality, our relationship to the pairs of opposites changes. Instead of trying to hold one and shun the other, we are able to transcend both, to experience them as two manifestations of a single reality. This experience wipes out many straight notions and thereby solves many problems, because many problems, as we saw in the last chapter, are rooted in the ego's conception of reality rather than in reality itself. For example, the whole mind-body problem that has stimulated such an outflow of straight prose becomes a problem only by thinking of it as such. The statement of the question limits the possible information one can get in an answer because it presupposes a meaningful distinction between the two phases of perceiving a single reality. Mind and body are really two expressions of the same phenomenon — just as waves and particles are two phases of expression of the entity called an electron.

Niels Bohr named the relationship between these two phases. He called it "complementarity." Bohr did not extend his understanding of an aspect of the nature of physical reality to all of human experience. But a contemporary chemist wrote in *Science* in 1971: "It is conceivable . . . , that the notion of complementarity offers a method of including both sensuous [i.e., experiential] and intellectual knowledge in a common frame of reference."[2] Deep thinking allows the direct experience of this single frame of reference — this one reality with its endlessly oscillating phases of wave/particle, light/dark, mind/body.

Unitive consciousness is the goal of all religions and philosophies of mind development. And one method of approaching the goal, all of these systems tell us, is by not trying to cling to one phase and avoid the other. Thus, Lao Tzu writes of the *Way of Life:*

> One who, preferring light,
> Prefers darkness also
> Is in himself an image of the world
> And, being an image of the world,
> Is continuously, endlessly
> The dwelling of creation.[3]

And in the *Bhagavad-Gita*, Krishna says:

> Feelings of heat and cold, pleasure and pain are caused by the contact of the senses with their objects. They come and they go, never lasting long. You must accept them.

> A serene spirit accepts pleasure and pain with an even mind and is unmoved by either. He alone is worthy of immortality.[4]

Probably, there are many valid techniques for achieving this kind of detachment. One method, a classical one, is to reach equilibrium by experiencing opposites simultaneously. Any quality can be neutralized by combining it with its opposite in equal strength; the principle applies to love and hate as well as to positron and electron. And, although the cancellation of opposites leads to a state designated mathematically by zero, the actual experience of this state is not of nothingness but of everythingness. For this reason, deep thinking leads also to:

3. Experience of infinity in its positive aspect

Whether we realize it or not, many of us have experienced infinity, but to ordinary consciousness the experience is intensely negative. I will give a personal example.

In 1964, when I was a senior in college, I took a large dose (40 milligrams) of psilocybin. At that time I did not understand psychedelics well enough to control them; nor did I know enough about set and setting to be able to shape the experience to the form I wanted it to take. I took the drug in a college dormitory room. Twenty minutes later, I suddenly began to experience striking visual illusions that became more and more kaleidoscopic. In one hour, my experience of reality had become completely fragmented, especially my intellectual experience, and since, as a good Harvard man, I was unable to detach myself from my intellect, the day became more and more unpleasant. The essence of this unpleasantness was symbolized by a recurring visual illusion and memory — the memory of sitting in barber chairs as a child, transfixed by the infinite regressions of mirrors facing each other. With a too-large dose of psilocybin, this same infinite regression burst in on every sense channel, and I had no way of orienting (or anchoring) myself in the ordinary reality in which I could commu-

nicate to others. My intellect was so affected that every time it produced a thought, it would automatically think about the thought,
think about thinking about the thought, and so on down the tun-
nel of mirrors. The more I tried to use my intellect to get me out of
the expanding confusion, the more dimensions the confusion as-
sumed.

I survived the storm, coming out of it after several hours with
only a bad headache. I have not made the same mistake again, and
I think I have profited greatly from the experience. For one thing,
it enabled me to see that all panic reactions to drugs (and, I suspect, to psychosis) in which patients think they are losing their
minds have at their heart this negative experience of infinity; having had the experience myself, I am now able to help others out of
it. Also, it adjusted my thinking by showing me starkly the inability of my intellect to deal with infinity, which, intuition tells me, is
surely an aspect of reality.

Just as we live in a universe where single realities express themselves in two opposite polarities or valences, so also we live in an
infinite universe where everything is relative. At every step in the
development of human consciousness, people have described limits to things, only to have those limits exploded by subsequent experience of things beyond. Indeed, the history of astronomy from
ancient Greece to the present is a continuing saga of an expanding
universe — expanding in the conceptions of human beings. And
try as we will with straight thinking to banish the notion of infinity, it keeps breaking in — in the heavens, in the subatomic world,
and, of course, in the barber shop. I think there is no need to add
that every religion uses the term *infinite* to describe its highest
conception, or that all mystics have seen infinity wherever they
looked. (Aldous Huxley took the title for his essay on mescaline
from the following line of William Blake: "If the doors of perception were cleansed, every thing would appear to man as it is —
infinite.")

The ego can see infinity only in its threatening aspect (that is,
threatening to the ego's limited world). Consequently, the ordinary

experience of infinity, if intense enough, is always accompanied by negative emotions and often by physical symptoms such as nausea (a very particular unpleasant sensation distinguished by its wavelike quality). To defend itself from these assaults, the intellect often tells us that the concept of infinity is meaningless or incomprehensible. And so it is, like every other mystery that can only be experienced directly. Only in the nonordinary consciousness of the lunar mind can we experience the looking-glass version of infinity in which the same perceptions evoke strongly positive reactions. The more we strive to extend and maintain awareness of our flashes of deep thinking, the more we can experience infinity positively, accept it, derive strength from it, and incorporate it consciously into our lives, thus decreasing the divergence between reality and our conceptions of it.

In this way, deep thinking leads us out of the predicament of straight thinking. As our conceptions come to fit reality better, action following from those conceptions produces the effects we want instead of the reverse. Rather than fighting negative manifestations of nature (and thereby making them assume worse forms), we are suddenly able to transform negative things into positive ones. Just as negative thinking is self-confirming, so is positive thinking; in sustained periods of lunar consciousness the sense that things are getting better and better is overwhelming — at least as powerful as the ego's conviction of imminent disaster. And a great deal of this optimism arises directly from one of the clearest messages coming across the intuitive channel: that there are no limits. The only limits we encounter in the world around us are those we first create in our imagination.

I have already written more in description of deep thinking than I intended to. I want now to discuss a number of conceptions I have come to as a result of episodic thinking in this way. If you can feel the truth of these conceptions, you will have a better idea of the process behind them than you could get from any amount of descriptive information.

1. Control of the autonomic nervous system

The autonomic nervous system is a well-known division of the general nervous system. It innervates all of the smooth (or involuntary) muscles, the heart muscles, and the gland cells throughout the body. It exerts major regulatory influences on many important structures, including the intrinsic muscles of the eye, the glands of the skin, and all of the cardiovascular, respiratory, digestive, endocrine, urinary, and reproductive systems. Neuroanatomists and neurophysiologists have long studied its two components, the sympathetic and parasympathetic systems, and much is known about how these systems connect to the organs they regulate. In some cases, the organs also receive fibers from the so-called voluntary motor pathway — a large system of nerves originating in the motor cortex of the brain and making connections in the spinal cord. Since the cortex (or outer covering) of the brain seems to participate in many of our "higher" mental functions, such as intellection, it makes sense that we can consciously will responses in our bodies by sending impulses along our voluntary motor pathways to our voluntary muscles. Breathing is the best example of a function with dual innervation: our respiration can be totally conscious or totally unconscious. In the first case, the voluntary nerves run things; in the second, the autonomic system carries the impulses.

We can think of the autonomic system as a more instinctive regulatory mechanism — one we share with many animals that lack our higher cortical centers. One of its qualities — the one responsible for its reputation as an involuntary system — is that it carries out its functions without our being aware of it. Moreover, if we try to will an autonomic response — say a change in our blood pressure — in the same way that we will a movement of our arm, we do not have much success. These facts have led many people to conclude that the autonomic nervous system has no direct connections to consciousness. But if we ask, To what kind of consciousness? the straightness of this conception becomes clear. For the autonomic nervous system seems to have very direct connections to every kind of consciousness but the ordinary one of the ego.

The most graphic illustration of this truth is a demonstration that has been made again and again in hypnotic subjects — one whose significance has been badly missed for decades by medical scientists. If a subject in a good trance is touched by a finger represented to him or her as a piece of hot metal, an authentic blister will develop at the point of contact. The blister is real. It is produced by autonomic innervation of superficial blood vessels. And this channel between the mind and the body is wide open whenever we are in an altered state of consciousness that focuses our awareness on something other than our ego and intellect.

Practitioners of meditation, especially students of yoga, have long known that autonomic responses can be brought under voluntary control. Adepts at yoga can suspend respiration for long intervals of time, effect drastic changes in heartbeat and circulation, and otherwise demonstrate that our internal functions are not beyond the reach of consciousness. In recent years, increasing numbers of Westerners, including physicians, have had a chance to observe these practices firsthand.

Texts on yoga are often vague about the techniques of achieving this kind of control (much of the information is transmitted orally from teacher to student), but from any survey of Eastern literature, three clues stand out. The first is that all of these accomplishments require relaxation, concentration, and practice. The second is that control of breathing is the key to the whole system. The third is that the first step to acquiring control of an autonomic response is to become aware of it. All of these suggestions are consistent with Western conceptions of neurophysiology.

Relaxation and concentration are means of detaching ourselves from ordinary consciousness, from that kind of consciousness where control of autonomic functions is not possible. In neurophysiological terms, this may mean suspending certain cortical activities, since the connections between the cortex and the autonomic system are not direct. Practice is the means by which potential neuronal pathways are developed, since repeated use of a circuit in the nervous system makes future use of that circuit easier.

The importance of breath control is that respiration is the one function in which the two motor pathways are in perfect potential balance. The theory behind yogic and other systems of disciplined breathing is that regular rhythms produced by the voluntary pathway will eventually be picked up by the involuntary pathway, and that once this sort of correspondence is established across the function of breathing, it spreads naturally to the other involuntary functions of heart rate, circulation, and so forth. It is significant that all Eastern and many Western systems of spiritual practice place great stress on breath control, also that the words for *spirit* and *breath* are identical in many Indo-European languages (including Sanskrit *[prana]*, Hebrew *[ruach]*, Greek *[pneuma]*, and Latin *[spiritus]*). Consider this excerpt from *Foundations of Tibetan Mysticism* by Lama Anagarika Govinda:

> The most important result of the practice of *"anapana-sati"* or "mindfulness with regard to breathing," is the realization that the process of breathing is the connecting link between conscious and subconscious . . . volitional and non-volitional functions, and therefore the most perfect expression of the nature of all life. Those exercises that lead to the deeper states of meditation . . . begin therefore with the observation and regulation of breath, which in this way is converted from an automatic or non-volitional function into a conscious one and, finally, into a medium of spiritual forces . . .
>
> Breath is the key to the mystery of life, to that of the body as well as to that of the spirit.[5]

Becoming aware of internal functions means paying attention to sensations we ignore in our ordinary waking state. As defined by neuroanatomists, the autonomic nervous system is purely motor, or efferent (that is, it carries impulses away from the brain to peripheral smooth muscles and glands). But it is well known that sensory nerves travel with this system, carrying information from the internal organs to the brain. These visceral afferent nerves, as they are called, are among the least understood components of the nervous system. We do not know what information they carry or how the brain integrates their messages into its infinitely complicated system of data processing. The experiential correlate of this lack of understanding is our own inability to feel what goes on inside our bodies except in the vaguest of ways. We are all aware of occasional sensations from our viscera, particularly if they are distended, but few of us can pinpoint the miscellaneous pains, twinges, and feelings that arise from inside our chests and abdomens. These visceral sensations are diffuse (that is, poorly localized), unclear as to quality, and of uncertain significance. Yet yogis say that with practiced concentration, one can greatly sharpen one's perception of these signals and that success in this practice leads automatically to greater autonomic control.

Working on this suggestion, a number of American researchers have begun to develop simple methods of teaching people to regulate internal functions. Known as "autonomic feedback control," these methods are all based on the principle of using external devices to augment internal signals so that they become perceptible without special practice. For example, blood pressure can be made continuously visible on an oscilloscope screen, or blood flow through an extremity can be shown on a moving graph. It turns out that if people in laboratories are provided with this sort of continuous feedback from an autonomic function to their external senses, they can quickly learn to modify the function. In this way, researchers in many parts of the country are demonstrating that heart rate, blood pressure, peripheral blood flow, and a variety of other functions thought to be beyond the reach of consciousness can be brought under voluntary control quite easily. These results have appeared in respectable journals* and are stimulating considerable interest among allopathic patients and practitioners alike.

The reason for the interest is obvious. Allopaths now have no methods for regulating autonomic functions with any specificity. Take the medications used to treat high blood pressure. The commonest variety of high blood pressure is called "essential hypertension" *(essential* being one of several words allopaths use to conceal their ignorance of the causes of specific ailments). It is a widely prevalent disease associated with serious complications over the course of years. Essential hypertension seems to be associated with a general increase in the tone of the sympathetic division of the autonomic nervous system, and allopathic treatment of the condition is often aimed at sabotaging this system, even to the point of surgically cutting sympathetic nerves. Unfortunately, these methods either do not alleviate the course of the disease much, or, if they are drastic enough, cause so many derangements of general sympathetic functioning that any decrease in blood pressure is offset by the appearance of other problems.† The finding that patients can be taught to lower blood pressure directly and specifically by the technique of autonomic feedback control opens a new and exciting frontier of treatment.

It is not necessary for people to know what they are doing when they learn to modify a function like heart rate or blood pressure; all they have to do is have feedback from the process to their senses. Furthermore, once they get a feel for the successful tech-

---

* See, for example, "Effects of Feedback and Reinforcement on the Control of Human Systolic Blood Pressure," by D. Shapiro, B. Tursky, E. Gershon, and M. Stern, *Science* 163 (7 February 1969), p. 588. Also, "Mind Over Body, Mind Over Mind," by Gay Luce and Erik Peper, *New York Times Magazine,* 12 September 1971, p. 34.

† Many antihypertensive drugs are marketed, and allopaths administer them to patients very frequently, but the ones that work do so many other things that they are dangerous — more dangerous than some illegal intoxicants. The other things are conveniently described as side effects in pharmaceutical advertising, although in practice the decrease in blood pressure is often the side effect in comparison with other changes.

nique, they can dispense with the external amplification and continue to practice anytime, anywhere. The success of these methods has led some researchers to conclude that Western technology is about to usher in an era of instant yoga and that yogis have been wasting their time.

I do not subscribe to these sentiments because it seems to me that yogis learn to do far more important things by their methods than gain control of particular autonomic processes. Autonomic feedback control is certainly important: if nothing else it shows us that common conceptions of the limits of conscious control are mistaken. But does it change our relationship to our unconscious minds? I am convinced that the unconscious mind stands in the same relationship to the autonomic nervous system as the conscious mind does to the voluntary motor pathway. *The problem, then, is not to learn to control the autonomic nervous system (since all of us are already doing that all the time); the problem is simply to open the channels between the conscious and the unconscious minds.*

We have seen that these channels are blocked in our ordinary waking state and are opened in altered states of consciousness like trances and highs. Autonomic feedback training bypasses these channels by routing an unconscious sensation through an external amplifying device. Doubtless this method has a very important place in specific clinical applications, but I do not think it will help us solve the general problem of establishing free interchange between our conscious and unconscious experience, between solar mind and lunar mind. In fact, by putting us in touch with certain possibilities of extended consciousness without teaching the general method of achieving and maintaining such control, it is open to the same criticisms that can be applied to drugs as means of reaching desired states of consciousness, including the inherent risk of dependence on something external and material to achieve something internal and nonmaterial. In short, although autonomic feedback training may help us treat our symptoms by ourselves and with natural methods (clearly steps in the right direction), it may not put us in touch with the causes of health and illness.*

2. The true causes of disease and the nature of nonallopathic healing

My intuitions about disease are: first, that its physical manifestations are mostly caused by nonmaterial factors, in particular by unnatural restraints placed on the unconscious mind; and second, that the limits to what human consciousness can cause in the physical body are far beyond where most of us imagine them.†

In suggesting that disease arises from the unconscious mind I am not denying the reality of the physical nervous system. Neurologists have very little to say about the correlations of unconscious experience with events in the brain (primarily because they, as the most mechanistic among allopaths, hesitate to use the concept of *mind* let alone that of *unconscious mind*). Neurological interest in the autonomic nervous system begins with the lower centers in the brain from which the fibers issue, not with the ultimate origins of the information carried by these fibers. Neuroanatomists, however, have traced the connections of these centers into a most interesting, poorly understood group of deep brain structures called the "limbic lobe." Is there any evidence that the limbic lobe is a physical correspondence of unconscious experience, as the cortex is the correspondence of conscious experience?

Here is some evidence that I find impressive. The limbic lobe of the brain is a primitive part of the nervous system in the sense that it is evolutionarily old. We share it with many lower animals. By contrast, the human cortex is a recent evolutionary development.

---

* Similarly, techniques that forcibly open channels to the unconscious without teaching us how to integrate conscious and unconscious energies may take us away from the goal rather than toward it. I am skeptical of many "new age" forms of psychotherapy for this reason.

† See my book *Health and Healing* (Boston: Houghton Mifflin, 1984) for development of these ideas.

In animals the structures that make up the limbic system are mainly concerned with the sense of smell; in man olfaction is a minor activity of the system, but the terms *rhinencephalon* and *smell-brain* are still used to designate the limbic structures. A great deal of evidence has been published suggesting that the limbic lobe is the seat of emotion and memory. (Odors are powerful releasers of emotions and unconscious memories.) Centers regulating eating and sexual behavior have been located in the rhinencephalon, as have pain and pleasure centers. Emotion, memory, smell, hunger, sex, pain, pleasure: all are experiences that have significant unconscious accompaniments. It seems very reasonable to me that the limbic system, as one physical correlate of the unconscious mind, is the origin of impulses that travel down the autonomic nerves to produce the organic changes of disease when the unconscious mind is cut off from waking awareness.

I mentioned earlier that essential hypertension is correlated with increased tone of the sympathetic nerves. Allopaths, seeing this correlate as a cause, cannot get to the root of the condition. The true cause is in the unconscious mind, which, denied access to consciousness, turns its energies downward. The neurological correlates of this process might be rhinencephalic discharges to the autonomic centers instead of to the cortex above; the physical effects on the body are as real as the blister on the arm of the hypnotized subject.

The unconscious mind turns against the body only when a higher part of the mind forces it to. Potential circuits exist for conducting unconscious impulses upward, as anyone knows who is aware of his daydreams and intuitions. (Again: the emphasis is on being *aware* of unconscious events.) It is the sealing of these channels from above that necessarily forces unbalanced unconscious energies down the autonomic nerves to produce negative physical effects.

The reasons for this sealing from above are known to all Freudians. The unconscious mind, on top of all its vital intrinsic functions, becomes the storehouse of everything the developing ego fears. Consequently, the ego attempts to block off the channels of communication to keep fears out of awareness. If we never learn to open the channels by disengaging our minds from ordinary consciousness (or, more accurately, by letting our nonordinary experiences into our waking awareness), we condemn ourselves to sickness and death.

These considerations form the theoretical basis of nonallopathic healing in all of its varied and sometimes bizarre forms. Earlier I wrote that allopathy was just one school of medicine, one way of doing things. Many others are in existence. Some, like osteopathy, are different from allopathy in name only; others are simple frauds. Few nonallopaths have any understanding of the reasons for their successes when they occur. Most are quite harmless in that they use noninjurious methods, unlike allopaths. Homeopaths, for instance, dispense tiny doses of drugs that reproduce the symptoms of illness rather than counteract them, in the hope that they will stimulate the body to react against the illness from within; a main virtue of homeopathy is that its drugs are given in minuscule amounts — too small to make anything worse.* Christian Scientists use no drugs or devices at all. Yet allopaths, as the lobbyists in control of medical legislation around the world, have made it difficult for nonallopaths to practice openly or profitably or to organize into professional power groups. A regrettable consequence is that it is difficult to get information about the effectiveness of nonallopathic healing.

Since leaving the world of allopathic practice, I have witnessed a number of impressive nonallopathic cures of serious allergies, infections, and toxic reactions. I have also studied reliable reports from colleagues and friends of nonallopathic cures of more dramatic illnesses, including cancer and life-threatening infections. Finally, I have watched a number of nonallopathic practitioners at work, among them faith healers and Native American medicine men. From this information, I have extracted a few simple princi-

* For a fuller discussion of homeopathy see *Health and Healing*, chapters 1–3.

ples that seem to me to underlie all successful nonallopathic practices and that are consistent with my intuitions about the true
causes of illness.

The power to heal, like the power to make ill, resides in the patient. An important clue to the nature of healing is the literal
meaning of the word: to make whole. The words *heal, whole,* and
holy are derived from a common root. And the concept of making
whole suggests to me the restoration of the natural state of openness between the conscious and unconscious minds — the reinte-
gration of consciousness, whose disintegration leads to illness in
the first place. The responsibility for this achievement rests ultimately with the sick person. An outside healer, however dramatic
his methods, can really do no more than two very simple things:
he can remove any obstacles to healing that are present, and he
can motivate the patient to get well.

When allopathic practitioners cure patients of illnesses they
do so in this same way, sometimes in spite of their methods, because, as we have seen, allopathic techniques can be obstacles
to healing. If a patient came to me, dependent on antibiotics,
with recurrent cycles of worsening infection, the first thing I
would do is remove the antibiotics. Similarly, the presence of foreign matter in an open wound constitutes an obstacle to healing,
as all surgeons know. Such obstacles need not be physical; anxiety
is a powerful obstacle that stands between many patients and
health.

In contrast to the allopathic fixation on symptoms, many nonallopathic healers ignore symptoms totally, and this difference
strikes me as very significant. Treatment of symptoms, however
sophisticated, focuses patients' attention on those symptoms, thus
reinforcing the anxiety and other negative feelings that helped
produce the symptoms in the first place. An important first step in
correct treatment is to distract the patient from the sensible evidence of his negative condition. Shamans and medicine men in
Indian societies are very adept at this sort of distraction; whether
they understand it or not, their elaborate dances and rituals, inde-

pendent of content, serve to focus the attention of patients away from their symptoms, thus greatly increasing the likelihood that healing will occur.

The second aspect of healing — motivating patients to heal themselves — is more subtle and, I suspect, not learnable in any conventional way. The essence of the process seems to be a kind of unconscious communication between healer and patient. It is especially noteworthy that healers get to be healers by being healed, in much the same way as psychoanalysts become psychoanalysts by being analyzed. I will have more to say about the nature of the interaction between healer and patient at the end of this chapter, when I discuss the reality of shared consciousness through the medium of the unconscious mind.

To the straight mind nonallopathic healing sounds mystical. Faith healing is held in contempt by most rational people, despite the abundant evidence of cures. What rational people fail to understand is that their systems require faith, too — faith in the intellect and the rational process. A supreme irony is that so-called rational methods require more faith than nonrational ones because they fly in the face of experience. I can illustrate this irony with a pharmacological example: the search for the nonaddicting narcotic.

Ever since widespread use of morphine as an analgesic began over a hundred years ago, pharmacologists have been obsessed with the search for a nonaddicting narcotic — one that would relieve pain but not cause dependence, produce euphoria but not addiction. By now that search has consumed untold amounts of time and money but it has been a consistent failure. A great many compounds have been invented and promoted as nonaddicting narcotics, among them heroin, meperidine (Demerol), hydromorphone (Dilaudid), and pentazocine (Talwin), but after longer or shorter periods of clinical use, their promoters have conceded that they are dependence producing. Hundreds and hundreds of molecular variations of constituents of opium have been concocted in laboratories and tested, but no matter how the molecules are twisted, the analgesic and dependence-producing properties cannot be separated.

Now, we saw earlier that neither analgesia nor drug dependence is a property of drugs. Morphine does not cause relief of pain any more than marijuana causes a high; it serves as a trigger for an altered state of consciousness in which pain is perceived differently than usual. Neither does morphine cause dependence; it becomes the object of dependent behavior arising from the misunderstanding of the cause-and-effect characteristic of materialism and straight thinking. In other words, analgesia and dependence are mixed up in people, not in drugs, and there is no point in trying to separate them by playing with molecules. The search for a nonaddicting narcotic is as fanciful as the search for gold that materialistic alchemists carried out in their laboratories. Furthermore, there is ample evidence that analgesia and dependence can be separated in one's consciousness. Anyone who learns to produce analgesia at will by self-hypnosis or meditation is an example.

Yet the search goes on. For years the National Institute of Mental Health has encouraged us to believe that its laboratories at Lexington, Kentucky, are on the verge of coming up with the magic molecule. What is this persistence but faith — blind faith in the ideas and methods of the intellect to solve a problem that is clearly insoluble as it is stated — faith that persists despite all the contrary evidence of actual experience. It seems to me that considerably less faith is required to go about learning to produce analgesia at will (through yogic practice, say) since the evidence of experience supports this approach. And this initial outlay of a smaller amount of faith is quickly rewarded by actual experiences that confirm the hypothesis.

In exactly the same way, faith healing, or healing by nonallopathic methods, seems to me to require considerably less faith than allopathic healing because it is consistent with intuitive knowledge of the causes of health and illness and because the evidence of actual experience supports it.

3. General anesthesia as an altered state of consciousness

As an allopathic physician and pharmacological researcher, I believed that general anesthesia was caused by a group of drugs called general anesthetics (including nitrous oxide, ether, chloroform, fluothane, and many other compounds). I no longer hold to that belief. Three facts are hard to explain if one believes that anesthetics cause anesthesia. First, although anesthesia has been around for over a hundred years and although millions of persons have been put into the state under close observation, no satisfactory theory of general anesthesia exists; doctors have no idea what these drugs do to the brain that accounts for the state. (A great many theories have been put forward, but none of them is supported by direct evidence.) Second, the chemicals that seem to cause anesthesia have nothing in common: they are a strikingly diverse group of compounds. Third, the state can be exactly reproduced without chemicals; in chapter 2 I told of seeing a Caesarean delivery performed without any drug, using only hypnosis to effect anesthesia.

When ether was first introduced, there were many reported failures to induce anesthesia with it. Today, a very powerful set exists among surgical patients that ether and other anesthetic gases will cause unconsciousness. But there are indications that persons in deep surgical anesthesia are, in fact, not unconscious. If, after recovery from an operation, a patient is hypnotized, he or she may be able to quote word for word conversations that went on while he was "asleep" on the operating table. (Many surgeons have learned, to their regret, that ill-advised remarks are recorded by the unconscious minds of anesthetized patients.)

All of these considerations suggest to me that general anesthesia is essentially an altered state of consciousness, not a pharmacological phenomenon. I also believe it to be a state of consciousness all of us could slip into at will if we knew how. This is not to say that the drugs do nothing. Their direct pharmacological actions (they interfere with neurological activity, particularly in the cortex of the brain) are an indirect push in the direction of the anesthetic state. In other words, there is a consistency of form between the pharmacological action of the drug and the state of consciousness.

General anesthesia looks to me like a state of intensely focused awareness with marked ego loss. It is a nonordinary experience, in which the unconscious mind takes over as the conscious mind suspends its activities. Persons unused to experiencing reality through their unconscious minds lose continuity of awareness on going into surgical anesthesia; on recovery they have no conscious memory of the experience (although the unconscious record can be recovered through hypnosis). But people who meditate well or have learned to use drugs to get closer to their unconscious minds can retain awareness even through deep surgical anesthesia. Their experience is nonordinary — for example, the operation may be perceived as in a dream — but it is continuous with the ordinary experience surrounding it.

American physicians who visited mainland China in 1971 reported that the traditional procedure of acupuncture (insertion of needles through the skin) is used successfully to produce general anesthesia for major surgery in modern Chinese hospitals. The needles would be no more causative of the phenomenon than our chemical anesthetics, but they are probably less dangerous. Let us hope that one day more of us will be able to shift into the state of consciousness in which pain ceases to hurt without any external devices or materials.

4. The necessity of a synthesis of Eastern and Western approaches to the mind

Throughout this book I have complained about the materialism of the West, its attachment to the intellect, and its blindness to nonordinary reality. I have also drawn constantly on the literature and experience of the East to document many of my hypotheses. I do not wish to be misunderstood as implying that the East, by itself, is closer to reality than the West.

By equating reality with material reality, Westerners deny themselves access to the true causes of physical phenomena, condemning themselves to the blind alley of straight thinking. Easterners tend to fall into the complementary trap of equating reality with nonmaterial reality, of dismissing the physical world as illusion. Consequently, they are no better able to change the physical world for the better and, in particular, are defenseless against the destructive power of Western materialism.

If I seem to stress Eastern themes, it is only because, as Westerners, we need them to offset our particular form of mental imbalance. But the goal I aim for is a total synthesis of Eastern and Western approaches to the mind. Consciousness is real. So is the physical nervous system. They are two expressions of the same underlying unitive phenomenon, and we must pay attention to both of them if we are to experience that phenomenon as a single reality.

The Eastern scientific approach to consciousness, with its emphasis on direct experience, shows us that the limits of our minds are not where we thought them to be. But this approach has also given rise to some very fanciful conceptions of the nervous system that simply do not agree with Western demonstrations of physical reality. Only by comparing the two approaches from a position of detached neutrality will we be able to weed out the errors in both in order to produce an amalgam of universal truth. A high priority in this comparison would be a thorough study of Eastern literature by people trained in the Western neurosciences. My own research in this direction convinces me that many exciting correspondences are waiting to be discovered.*

* The most interesting possibility is the use of technologies like PET (positron emission tomography) scans of living brains to determine correlations between states of consciousness and central nervous system activity. Such studies have demonstrated differences between brain activity of experienced meditators and nonmeditators in response to various kinds of stimulation.

Here is a quick example. I wrote earlier that children (and some adults) often have unusual experiences at the point of falling asleep, including out-of-body experiences. We in the West know that the brain is in a unique electrophysiological state at this transition point. Brain waves are distinct between waking and sleeping, and the "seizure threshold" dips to a low point at this time (that is, it is easiest to produce a convulsion). In the light of this knowledge, consider a line from a Hindu text that is 4,000 years old, in which a god (Shiva) reveals to a goddess 112 ways of achieving superconsciousness. Method number fifty has been translated as follows: "At the point of sleep when sleep has not yet come and external wakefulness vanishes, at this point *being* is revealed."[6]

Unfortunately, most Western neuroscientists look down their noses at the Eastern literature of consciousness, failing to see its relevance. And the few who do wake up to it become so excited that, more often than not, they disown their Western heritage and run off to the Himalayas to become Easterners. I hope we will begin to see a new breed of students of the mind who realize the complementary nature of the two approaches and the necessity of working toward a synthesis. As the great teachers have said over and over, the truth is always in the middle.

5. Positive paranoia

Paranoia — a common experience in the drug subculture and elsewhere — is not simple fear. Rather it is the tendency to see external events and things forming patterns that appear to be inimical. It is important to distinguish between the two components of paranoia — the seeing of patterns and the negative interpretation of them — something few people bother to do. What most of us (including most psychiatrists) call paranoia is really negative paranoia — one side of a mental state that is in itself neutral. When we understand this principle (that is, when we get out of the straight perception), we open ourselves to the possibility of understanding and experiencing positive paranoia.

The pattern-forming tendency (I am tempted to call it an ability) is an intrinsic function of the unconscious mind.* When we allow it to impose itself on our perceptions, we see relationships between things that are not apparent to other people (at least, not to other people using their minds in straight ways). Clinical psychologists can easily document this ability on their Rorschach (inkblot) tests, where it is scored as the "W-tendency," W standing for "whole." A person with a strong W-tendency will attempt to fit all of the fragmented parts of an inkblot into one integrated whole. In the early cards of the standard ten-card series, it is not hard to account for all the markings (one blot looks very much like a butterfly, for instance), but the later cards are as fragmented as Jackson Pollock paintings. A person with a strong W-tendency has a lot of trouble accounting for all the pieces of these blots, and his difficulty will be apparent to a trained psychologist. The W-tendency correlates well with a tendency to paranoia.

A full-blown episode of negative paranoia can be very frightening for everyone concerned. When a person is acutely paranoid, he can fit every piece of sense data into his pattern. Thus everything that happens, anything that anyone does to help is interpreted as further evidence of a "conspiracy against me." Allopathically conditioned psychiatrists can only think of this reaction as a symptom to be counteracted, as with sedation.

But anyone who reads firsthand accounts of mystic experience or flashes of enlightenment must be struck by the underlying identity with negative paranoia. Mystics of all centuries have experienced the entire phenomenal world as a radially symmetrical pattern, its center coinciding with the center of focused consciousness. But they have interpreted the experience positively, if not

---

* When we are open to the unconscious, patterns may come through to us visually, either in the mind's eye or as illusions projected onto incoming visual signals. Many of these patterns assume archetypal forms that have been used as sacred and secular motifs by widely separated civilizations. In trances or hallucinogen-induced states, psychiatric patients sometimes describe radially symmetrical patterns identical with ancient Hindu mandalas, even though they have never seen mandalas with their conscious minds. I have often seen similar patterns on surfaces after taking mescaline and LSD.

with ineffable joy. Mystical experience is the mirror image of negative paranoia. And the two are the two complementary expressions of a single experience, that of the center of a pattern.

Psychologists in the Haight-Ashbury Research Project of Mount Zion Hospital's Department of Psychiatry (an NIMH-funded project) have turned up cases of what they call "benign paranoia": young members of the San Francisco drug subculture who had strong W-tendencies on Rorschach tests but who seemed to feel that "the universe is a conspiracy organized for my benefit." The researchers were impressed that these persons seemed to function well in their communities even though they looked unhealthy by the standard criteria of psychological testing.

The ability to see patterns, far from being a psychological weakness to be treated, is a vital capacity of the unconscious mind that must be developed and allowed to interact with our conscious perceptions. When nonordinary experience is not allowed into ordinary awareness it breaks through in destructive, negative ways such as episodes of negative paranoia. The goal should not be to make negative paranoia go away but to turn it into a source of psychological strength and joy. The first step toward that goal is to exchange the straight conception of paranoia for the deep one — to look at the positive potential of a seemingly negative phenomenon.

6. Positive neurosis

Neurosis is simply the negative experience of ambivalence. Therapists' offices are filled with persons who have been unable (fortunately) to seal off completely the channels to their unconscious minds. But in their continuing attachment to ego-centered consciousness they cannot accept their own ambivalent nature. For example, the ego cannot understand that it is possible to love and hate someone simultaneously or that these two reactions are complementary expressions of a single phenomenon. In its efforts to disown the negative phase, the ego struggles more and more to bury it in the unconscious, thus perpetuating the conflict. Symptomatic neurotics are those whose discouragement at this straight predicament begins to interfere with their functioning in the world.

The solution is not to reinforce the ego so that it can withstand the conflict but to flip neurosis into its positive phase. Ambivalence, as we have noted, is in the nature of things. Acceptance of the negative or destructive components of one's own personality leads to the formation of an integrated personality, a whole consciousness. The most creatively talented people in our society are usually also the most neurotic. Many of them have discovered in their own experience that neurosis is a source of energy: that is, the energy that leads to creative production is the same energy that goes more often into the maintenance of neurotic behavior (including habitual use of drugs). Perhaps everyone is potentially a creative genius; neurotics have taken one step toward realization of that potential. The next step comes with a change in point of view of the process of neurosis.

7. Positive psychosis

Psychotics are persons whose nonordinary experience is exceptionally strong. If they have not integrated this experience into conscious awareness (or so repressed it that it causes physical illness), it takes very negative mental forms. But every psychotic may be a potential sage or healer and to the extent that negative psychotics are burdens to society, to that extent can positive psychotics be assets. (In Native American societies, what we might call psychotic experience in adolescence is a sign that the individual is chosen as a future shaman.) To effect this transformation we must remove obstacles to the change (such as antipsychotic drugs and most institutional psychiatry) and bring patients into contact with healed compatriots — that is, with persons who have themselves made the transformation. Such people exist; we simply must allow psychotics to seek them out and learn from them.

The National Institute of Mental Health defines schizophrenia as the nation's number one mental-health priority. But in its totally straight approach, it has stated the problem in an insoluble way. Schizophrenia is indeed incurable in allopathic terms because it cannot be made to go away. (Once one realizes that the single authorized version of reality psychiatrists promote with their talk of "reality testing" is a fiction, there is no going back.) Much of NIMH's efforts have been directed toward a fantastic goal: the discovery of the biochemical cause of psychosis, an effort that has been a dismal failure for twenty years now. Despite expenditures of enormous amounts of money and time and the discovery, one after the other, of "promising" biochemical correlates of schizophrenia, psychosis is bigger than ever and our power to change it is no greater than it was when NIMH started pouring our tax money down the research drain many years ago. Even if disorders of body chemistry are found to correlate well with schizophrenia (and most correlates found so far turn out not to be specific to the condition), it makes much more sense to see them as expressions of disorders of consciousness rather than the reverse. If it sticks to its present course, NIMH will be the last institution in America to recognize the positive potential of psychosis — a potential so overwhelming that I am almost tempted to call psychotics the evolutionary vanguard of our species. They possess the secret of changing reality by changing the mind; if they can learn to use that talent for positive ends, there are no limits to what they can accomplish.

8. The reality of shared consciousness

C. G. Jung's model of a collective unconscious is extremely useful. It appears that at some level of the unconscious we pass beyond personal awareness into a universal awareness unlimited by time and space. Most of us may think we never experience such a thing, but it may be that we simply never pay attention to it. I am convinced it happens.

Read carefully this example from the same narrative quoted earlier of a Peruvian youth, kidnapped by Amazonian Indians who
used the hallucinogenic drink called *ayahuasca*. The young man
took the drug many times with the tribe and always had intense visions in which jungle animals played prominent roles. Here is his
report of an *ayahuasca* session called by the chief, who was about
to die:

It was a select group of twelve that went to the secluded glade in the
forest. It included some of the older men and several of the best
hunters. The rituals and chants were similar to previous occasions,
perhaps a little more elaborate. From the preparatory chants of the
fragrant smoke and evocation of the spirit of the *honi xuma* [i.e., of
the vine that provides the drug] it was evident that Chief Xumu was
attempting in this session to fix in my consciousness all the important or essential circumstances of their tribal life. There seemed to
be an intense feeling of rapport among the group, all dedicated to
the purpose of the old man.

I was aware of the fragile hand that poured the magic fluid and
passed the cups around to each. We drank in unison and settled into
a quiet reverie of joint communion, savoring the fragrant smoke in
the stillness of the silent forest. A quiet chant held our conscious
thoughts together as the potion took effect. A second cup was passed
to intensify the reaction.

Color visions, indefinite in form, began to evolve into immense
vistas of enchanting beauty. Soon subtle but evocative chants led by
the chief took control of the progression of our visions. Embellish-
ments to both the chants and the visions came from the participants.

Soon the procession of animals began, starting with the jungle
cats. Some of these I had not seen before. There was a tawny puma,
several varieties of the smaller spotted ocelot, then a giant rosetta-
spotted jaguar. A murmur from the assembly indicated recognition.
This tremendous animal shuffled along with head hanging down,
mouth open and tongue lolling out. Hideous, large teeth filled the
open mouth. An instant change of demeanor to vicious alertness
caused a tremor to run through the circle of phantom-viewers.

From a memory recess in my brain there emerged with the stimulation of the cats an experience from my past. On a trip to the Rio Putumayo a year before coming to the Jurua to cut *caucho* [rubber], I had come face to face on a forest path with a rare black jaguar. It had been a terrifying experience, but I had dominated the flashing eyes of the beast and we had gone our separate ways without violence.

This mighty animal now intruded on our visions and a shudder passed through us all. As before, the demon of the forest went on his way. Other animals, snakes, birds passed in review, each with some significant characteristic important to the Huni Kui [the tribe] in dominating the forest.

Then came scenes of combat with the hated enemy, the Guacamayos . . . a procession of the feared white-robed and hooded Bolanxos, and encounters with Kariwa and Kiruana, the hated invading rubber cutters. In one vision a village was in flames, the people scattering in panic into the forest. Here Xumu, then a much younger man, killed a rubber cutter in violent hand-to-hand fighting.

Scenes in the new village, where we now lived, gradually brought the visions to an end. We awoke to shafting sunlight and morning bird song penetrating both to our consciousness and to the place of our visions.

As I have explained before, it is impossible to describe satisfactorily the content and depth of feeling that captures the mind. During the visions I was aware within myself of a great feeling of empathy for these people in their struggle to dominate the forces of nature for their daily living and to defend themselves against their enemies.

A calabash of thick fruit gruel passed around by one of the guards restored our bodily sensations to the daily world of our existence, and in a subdued mood we returned to the village. Everyone seemed aware of the source of the black jaguar sequence of visions. It left a strong impression on them and resulted in my being given the name Ino Moxo, Black Panther.[7]

Evidently, these Indians experience the collective unconscious as an immediate reality, not just as an intellectual construct. It is significant that this experience of shared consciousness holds a most important place in the society. In fact, as a sacramental ritual, it is the basis of tribal unity because it proves and confirms the supposition that every person in the tribe is the same as every other person in the most fundamental way. I believe also that this kind of unconscious communication is the channel through which the wholeness of a healer can be transmitted to a sick person.

Of course, the drug does not cause this effect. It is a natural capacity of man's unconscious mind. Nor is there anything special about these Indians, except their relative lack of attachment to ego and intellect. Not only do I think each of us can share consciousness, I think all of us are already doing it all the time. We do not have to learn to be telepathic; we just have to notice that we already are by letting telepathic events into our waking awareness.

Extrasensory perceptions are not unusual talents possessed by specially gifted individuals. They are normal unconscious events, and scientists who attempt to document them by laboratory experiments will never get to experience them directly. Lama Govinda, drawing on his experience as a member of a Tibetan Buddhist order, says of Tibetans:

> . . . [They] rely a great deal on their dream consciousness, and they are seldom proved wrong in their judgment.
> Besides dreams they have many other methods of contacting the deeper layers of their mind: meditation, trance, certain forms of oracles, and various natural and "supernatural" (psychic) portents. All these methods have been tried out for millenniums, and their results have been found sufficiently satisfactory to guide people in their daily life. Tibetans would be greatly surprised if one would doubt these facts, which are matters of practical experience and have nothing to do with beliefs or theories. To them the attempts of modern psychologists, who try to "prove" extrasensory perception by scientific methods, would appear crude and laughable: one might just as well try to prove the existence of light which is visible to all but the blind. The circumstances under which these modern experiments are carried out are in themselves the greatest hindrance to their success. In their attempt at "objectivity" they exclude the emotional and

the spiritually directive elements of the human mind, without which no state of real absorption or concentration can be created. Their very attitude bars the doors of psychic perception.[8]

Because awareness of shared consciousness requires relaxation, concentration, and detachment from the ordinary activities of the ego, it comes naturally with any practice in these directions. Patanjali devoted a whole section of his yoga aphorisms to a listing of the various psychic powers one may obtain through concentration, but he warned that students who pursue these powers as ends in themselves will not attain the highest states of consciousness.

That communication of this sort exists is really no more remarkable than the fact that intuition exists. The rational mind cannot provide any explanation for intuition any more than it can for other extrasensory phenomena. Anyone who has learned to pay attention to and trust his or her intuitions knows that the mind contains a source of information about reality quite apart from the senses. In fact, paying attention to intuitions is one way of becoming aware of related unconscious activities.

I believe that the visual imagination is another doorway to the collective unconscious. Practice at seeing with the mind's eye puts us more in touch with the level of the unconscious that is no longer purely personal. Hence the visionary is able to receive communications that others are not aware of. A professor of humanities wrote in the *New York Times:*

> If you went around in England in 1770 asking people how it felt to be living in an age of Industrial Revolution, most people would not know what you were talking about. But if you went to see the "lunatic" William Blake living in obscurity, he would tell you about the meaning of the great cultural transformation . . . From a few eighteenth century brick kilns he was able to extrapolate imaginatively the complete transformation of human society.
>
> Imaginative artists like Blake can understand the collective condition of society because the imagination is itself the opening to the

collective unconscious; and precisely because this consciousness is collective, imaginative people can think the same thought at the same time even though they are separated by ordinary space.[9]

Telepathy is nothing other than thinking the same thoughts at the same time others are thinking them — something all of us are doing all the time at a level of our unconscious experience most of us are not aware of. Become aware of it and you become telepathic automatically. Doubtless this experience also has a physical correlate in the brain. My own hunch is that the visual cortex (in the occipital lobes of the brain at the back of the head) is the neurological apparatus that mediates this function when it is not occupied with the normal processing of visual data from the eyes (that is, when we learn to withdraw attention from incoming visual signals). And perhaps the people best qualified to teach us about this system are not neurophysiologists but Indians who regularly go off into forests to see the same visions simultaneously.

It is time to return to the here and now of our own society with all of its anxieties about drugs that appear to affect the mind. I have introduced this discussion of solar mind and lunar mind, of straight versus deep thinking, for a specific purpose: to make it possible for us to understand why everything done in the name of stopping the drug problem only makes it worse and why changes in our basic conceptions must come about before anything will start to get better. Our trip to the moon has been brief and tantalizing. Readers who wish to follow up some of the ideas in this chapter should see Suggested Reading on page 191, but they should bear in mind that the best source of information is the direct experience of their own inner states.

8. The Only Solution to the Drug Problem

A
S SOON AS WE UNDERSTAND the difference between straight and deep thinking we can see at once that all of our approaches to social problems associated with drugs are based in the former. Indeed, the very notion of a drug problem is straight because it implies that drugs are causative of negative behavior connected with their use.

Instead of beating to death our social programs aimed at curbing drug abuse, I will simply mention certain conceptions that seem to me to be representative. For example, the idea that disliked drugs can be forced out of existence is typical of a way of thinking that has dominated our minds since the beginning of the twentieth century. Despite the fact that action based on this premise has been consistently correlated with increasing prevalence of drug use and increasing negativity of drug use, the premise is still used as the basis of action. Many Americans, including many legislators and government executives, continue to dream that marijuana and narcotics can be made to vanish by sealing off borders, eradicating hemp and coca plants, paying foreign governments not to grow opium, and so on. And when, in response to these actions, drug use becomes greater and worse, the only thing such people can see to do is to redouble their efforts. Here once again is the familiar vicious cycle. It is perfectly logical that straight thinking on the part of society gets it into the same predicament that besets an individual who thinks that way. Interestingly enough, many analysts of social processes see this vicious cycle in other areas of American life, although they do not connect it with a general error of thinking. For example, Jay W. Forrester, a professor of management at the Massachusetts Institute of Technology, wrote in 1971:

> The nation exhibits a growing sense of futility as it repeatedly attacks deficiencies in our social system while the symptoms continue to worsen. Legislation is debated and passed with great promise and hope. But many programs prove to be ineffective. Results often seem unrelated to those expected when the programs were planned. At times programs cause exactly the reverse of desired results . . .
> . . . In fact a downward spiral develops in which the presumed solution makes the difficulty worse and thereby causes a redoubling of the presumed solution.[1]

Like the fantasy that drugs can be made to go away, the idea that people who want drugs can be discouraged from using them is an impossible dream that gets us nowhere except in worse trouble. Despite Draconian penalties for possession of marijuana and heroin, everyone who has wanted to use these drugs has done so over the years. Many persons, especially young ones, have wanted to use these drugs primarily because society threatens such punishments. ("If they tell us it's that bad, there must be something to it.") I would extend these comments to all of our criminal legislation on drugs. It has become apparent to many (including to many law-enforcement officers) that criminal law is simply not the appropriate means to use to affect drug taking in our society — a lesson that might have been learned from the failure of Prohibition. This does not mean that it is any better to try for the same unrealistic goals through education instead. "The drug problem must be solved by education, not law enforcement" has become a familiar slogan in enlightened circles, but in my experience the people who use it mean that educators are to take over the job of keeping young people from using disapproved drugs by scaring them in more sophisticated ways than policemen can. That would not be a real change.

In fact, all of the other liberal solutions to the problem seem to me just as straight as, and in some cases worse than, the simple-minded police approach. Methadone maintenance for heroin addicts is shockingly off the mark. Instead of showing heroin users how to get high without drugs, it gives them drugs without highs — exactly the wrong direction in which to change things. Not surprisingly, the developers and promoters of methadone maintenance hold grossly materialistic conceptions of addiction.*

The "Twelve Step" method seems to me equally flawed, although it may be useful at present in the absence of anything better. It first appeared in Alcoholics Anonymous. Twelve-step programs demand complete abstinence from drugs using the techniques of group support and encounter therapy to help addicts remain abstinent. Underlying this approach are some very negative conceptions: that drug use is a sickness, that addicts have a fatal weakness that makes them susceptible to addiction, that they will always have this weakness, and, therefore, that total forced abstinence is the only solution. Such programs claim great success, but they are very self-selective, and only a tiny percentage of all drug users can participate. Furthermore, people who succeed are often unable to become independent of the program (that is, they transfer their addiction from drugs to the program); many become program administrators or set up similar groups in other parts of the country. Some are fanatical propagandists, and I have seen them do enormous harm at public drug forums where they inflame anxiety by recounting the horrors of the drugs that "caused" all their problems. Though they abstain from the object of their desire, they have done nothing about the real cause of

* Dr. Vincent Dole is an example. A 1971 Ford Foundation paper on the state of knowledge of heroin said: "Dr. Vincent Dole has suggested that an addict may have an underlying neurological vulnerability to addiction that is triggered by opiate use. More recently, he has stated opiate use may trigger a metabolic change which causes the body to crave opiates thereafter. Dole is not optimistic about the possibilities of research on this question of metabolic change, however. He has said that it is probably not a researchable question given the present state of the pharmacological art, because of the lack of testable hypotheses that might explain it."

their addictive behavior, which was the confusion of the drug with a vital experience, the confusion of the outward form with the inner contents. Twelve-step programs do not change addicts' conceptions for the better; they merely reinforce the usual error of thinking. Krishna sums up this situation neatly in the *Bhagavad-Gita:*

> The abstinent run away from what they desire
> But carry their desires with them:
> When a man enters Reality,
> He leaves his desires behind him.[2]

I will stick to my statement that *all* of our efforts to solve social problems associated with drugs are based in straight thinking and are, therefore, making things worse instead of better. I cannot help feeling that what we are now doing in the name of stopping the drug problem *is* the drug problem. In many states and communities I have visited over the past three years, persons concerned with drug abuse are under enormous pressure to do something, but no one seems to know what to do. It has become routine to hold forums about drugs, appropriate more funds for law enforcement and education, conduct surveys in schools to determine the incidence of use, and issue reassurances that the problem is "not as big as we imagined." But everyone can see that use has never been greater and is growing at an accelerating rate. What can we do?

In the very first paragraph of this book I said that I was not presenting a program for social reform but rather "the germ of a new way of thinking about drugs and consciousness — a way that creates possibilities for solving a problem . . ." I will not recommend specific actions. But I can say what will certainly not work.*

---

* For example, even if the common illegal drugs could be made to vanish, users would simply find other substances (active placebos) to trigger highs, just as marijuana smokers will resort to nutmeg when they are confined to prisons where marijuana is unobtainable. Many spices can be used for this purpose as well as a great many native plants. In general, the substances people use when they are cut off from their usual drugs are more toxic than the ones they normally take.

And, more importantly, I can point out where the real solutions lie.

The underlying premise of this whole book has been that non-material factors cause material effects. A deduction from this premise is that the drug problem is an effect of conceptions about drugs and that it can only be solved by changing those conceptual models. Professor Forrester has also written:

> Each of us uses models constantly. Every person in his private life and in his business life instinctively uses models for decision making. The mental image of the world around you which you carry in your head is a model. One does not have a city or a government or a country in his head. He has only selected concepts and relationships which he uses to represent the real system. A mental image is a model. All of our decisions are taken on the basis of models. All of our laws are passed on the basis of models. All executive actions are taken on the basis of models. The question is not to use or ignore models. The question is only a choice among alternative models.[3]

Until the models that produce the current laws, decisions, and actions about drugs change, nothing about drugs will change, hence the uselessness of pressing for legal reform as a means of solving the drug problem. Counterproductive laws against possession and sale of drugs are not causes of problems; they are symptoms of problems at the level of conceptions, of mental images, just as physical symptoms of illness are effects of mental states. We saw earlier that action directed against symptoms tends to intensify symptoms. For this reason, I have never worked for repeal of any drug laws. Clearly, no drug should be illegal, but the way to reach that ideal state is not merely by fighting specific laws.* Simi-

---

* In May 1971 I was invited to testify before the National Commission on Marijuana and Drug Abuse. I explained my views on altered states of consciousness, the need to get high, and the indirect relationship of drugs to highs. In conclusion I said:

   ... I oppose the legalization of marijuana to the extent that it is represented as a way of improving the dreadful state we are in with regard to all drugs. The drug problem is a manifestation of useless ways of thinking at all levels of society — among

larly, there is no point in venting our frustration against law-enforcement officers or legislators. Enforcement officers simply enforce laws on the books and will continue to do so; they did not put the laws on the books — we did. And even though our legislators enacted those laws, we gave them the power to express our collective will in laws. We have the legislatures we deserve and always will. It is *our* conceptions that must change.

The ways of thinking about drugs contained in this book are new models that can serve us better. I have tried to show that they explain observable data and experience better than existing models. Now, I will try to show how they create possibilities for social change.

I have argued that every human being is born with an innate drive to experience altered states of consciousness periodically — in particular to learn how to get away from ordinary ego-centered consciousness. I have also explained my intuition that this drive is a most important factor in our evolution, both as individuals and as a species. Nonordinary experiences are vital to us because they are expressions of our unconscious minds, and the integration of conscious and unconscious experience is the key to life, health, spiritual development, and the fullest use of our nervous systems. By instilling fear and guilt about altered states of consciousness into our children, we force this drive underground, guaranteeing that it will be expressed in antisocial ways.

I have repeatedly stressed that drugs are merely means to achieve states of nonordinary awareness and must not be con-

---

users of drugs as well as non-users. Until those ways of thinking change, all the factors producing the problem will continue to produce it, even though the specific forms of it may change. If marijuana is legalized, no real change will occur. Just as many young people will be involved with the law in just as many bad ways; there will be just as much public clamor for changes in drug laws — probably for legalization of hallucinogens and heroin; just as many people will be using drugs in unintelligent ways; and, worst of all, just as many people will be missing out on the realization of the positive development of consciousness to higher levels. The only change will be that the liberals who advocate legalization will be able to sleep easier at night, thinking they have done something to make things better, and I would view that as a retrogressive step.

fused with the experiences themselves. They have the capacity to trigger highs; they do not contain highs. Moreover, the experiences they trigger are essentially no different from experiences triggered by more natural means. Many of the dangers attributed to drugs have no basis in fact but arise entirely from our own fears, which lead us to interpret our perceptions in certain ways and to see drugs as causes of the behavior they are merely correlated with. The real risk of using drugs as the primary method of altering consciousness is in their tendency to reinforce an illusory view of cause and effect that makes it ultimately harder to learn how to maintain highs without dependence on the material world. But we saw also that this risk can be contained by making use of principles employed by Amazonian Indians: in particular, by using natural drugs in natural ways, surrounding their use with ritual, relying on the supervision of experts qualified by their own experience, and applying the states of consciousness to positive ends, such as developing conscious awareness of unconscious events.

With these conceptions instead of old ones, and using deep thinking instead of straight thinking, what conclusions can we come to about how society might proceed? Straight thinking looks always to the negative side of things, which, in the case of drugs, is easy enough to see. If we are to begin to change things, we must start to look for the positive potential underneath negative experiences, for the secret of realizing such potential is first to have a clear mental image of it. Therefore, I will insist that we accept the fact that drugs — intelligently used as tools to enter other states of consciousness — are potentially beneficial. I and many of my friends would never have thought about meditation, higher levels of consciousness, or spiritual matters if we had not been in contact with the drug subculture and had not been through phases of meaningful use of marijuana and psychedelics.

In October 1970 I attended a study group meeting titled "A Review of the Biomedical Effects of Marijuana on Man in the Military Environment," sponsored by the Federation of American Societies of Experimental Biology at the request of the Life Sciences Division of the Army Research Office. The participants were mostly straight-thinking researchers, all well-known experts in the field. One, a medical doctor famous for his investigations of THC in animals and humans, ridiculed the suggestion that marijuana users might have legitimate insights into the nature of reality. Many of the ideas presented in the two previous chapters are insights (or intuitions) I first became aware of when I was high on marijuana. I would be happy to defend them in public discussion with any marijuana expert who does not know the positive potential of the drug from his own experience.

As soon as we begin to understand that drugs have a positive side that can be developed, we no longer need try to make drugs go away, which, as we have seen, makes them more of a problem. For drugs are perfect examples of the ambivalence of external things. They are potential keys to better ways of using the mind; they are also potential traps that can keep us from using our minds in better ways. Which potential becomes reality is entirely up to us because it depends entirely on which side we tend to look at in forming our conceptions. As long as we continue to ridicule the possibility that drugs can help us, we have no chance of making them less harmful to us. If we rely on our intellects and senses, we formulate inductive hypotheses based on the negative appearances of drugs and come up with the same straight ideas that have failed us consistently throughout the century. If we can even start to move in the direction of relying on intuition and experience to discover the positive potential of drugs, the drug problem will automatically begin to recede. I maintain that this latter approach is the only realistic course of action for our society; there is no other way.

Once we accept the general premise, it seems to me that our actions must be directed toward two specific goals: (1) encouragement of people who wish to use drugs to use them intelligently for their own good and thereby for the good of society; and (2) encouragement of people to progress beyond drugs to better methods of altering consciousness. Who is to do the encouraging? Clearly, all of us must work toward these ends, not just educators, government officials, or legal and medical professionals. Parents and teachers must do a large part of the job, but the effort will have to be truly collective. And in this effort, it will be wise to remember that our energies go farthest in changing our own thinking. Our own conceptions must change before we can effectively change those of other people.

Because so much of the process I envision will go on in individuals, I cannot give specifics that will apply to all of us. But I can give examples of things I would like to see come about as steps in the right direction.

I would like to see all people interested in the drug problem begin to seek out people who actually use drugs to learn from them about their experiences. They are easy to find and usually pleased to be asked what their highs are like. Parents should ask their children to tell about the positive aspects of drugs rather than lecture them about the negative ones and should look for similarities to their own episodes of nonordinary consciousness. Psychiatrists should *listen* to what their patients say about drug experiences; patients often know more about the workings of the unconscious mind from direct experience than doctors do from their intellects. Teachers should try to learn from students who know more about the subject than they do. In these ways, we will come to have better information than what we now get from experts who do not know from their own experience what they are talking about.

I would like to see all of us who use legal drugs — caffeine, nicotine, alcohol — to begin seeing these substances for the drugs they are and their habitual use for the addictions they are. Users of these strong legal drugs must try to understand that they are not really different from users of illegal substances.

I hope that users of illegal drugs will begin to come forward to volunteer information they have gathered about states of consciousness and techniques they have discovered for using drugs to best advantage. Users must come to realize that the present attitude of society toward them is as much due to their own negative thinking as to that of nonusers. Straight mentality is not a habit peculiar to nonusers of illegal drugs.

I would like to see social programs aimed against drug abuse begin to make use of persons who have learned how to use drugs intelligently. These persons will be our shamans; they are the only people who will ever be able to teach our children how to live in a world containing drugs and not get hurt by them.

I want to see the emergence of a new science of consciousness built up by free-thinking refugees from the traditional fields now stifled by materialism: the neurosciences, computer sciences, psychology, psychiatry, and so on. Consciousness itself must be the central focus of this endeavor, with the direct information of experience valued as much as intellectual knowledge and the vast body of Eastern psychological literature given as much attention as the Western.*

I hope that religious organizations in this country will begin to understand that highs triggered by drugs may be more relevant to spiritual development than appearances of spirituality on Sunday mornings. If religious leaders disapprove of the use of drugs, then they had better look to their own mystic traditions for information on alternative methods to reach the same states of consciousness.

I want to encourage those who have had psychotic experiences to look to the positive side of this change; to resist the negative conceptions of their minds offered to them by psychiatrists and society at large; and to look to their fellow psychotics for strength and knowledge of how to control and use their expanding consciousness for positive ends.

All of us, I hope, will begin knowing materialism for what it is so that we can eliminate it from our science and our systems of

---

* This development has already started. Such movements as Humanistic Psychology and Transpersonal Psychology are well under way in the right direction. The Menninger Foundation in Topeka, Kansas, has held numerous annual conferences on the voluntary control of internal states. And the University of Arizona has put on several large conferences on consciousness.

medicine, law, and government. Above all, we must come to understand the value of nonordinary experience — to feel grateful for it rather than guilty about it — so that we can encourage our children to express it rather than hide it.

These changes in point of view cannot happen overnight, for they require acceptance of painful truths: that children daydreaming in class, for example, might be using their minds much more profitably than children paying attention;* that psychotic patients may be in a better position to understand and experience reality than the psychiatric authorities who dose them with antipsychotic medications. But we can take the first step toward these goals at once: learning to tolerate nonordinary experience in others requires nothing more than acceptance of it in one's own life. Every person who becomes less anxious and more open about his or her own altered states of consciousness will have done something concrete to help solve the drug problem — in fact, will have done the only thing that can possibly help.

In conclusion, I have nothing more to say than this: drugs are with us to stay. Fight them and they will grow ever more destructive. Accept them and they can be turned into nonharmful, even beneficial forces.

---

* An elementary-school teacher in the Midwest once told me that she had a problem with a creative boy who daydreamed in class constantly. If she bothered him too much he would force her to excuse him by causing his temperature to go up so that she would have to send him to the school nurse. Although both teacher and nurse knew that the boy could produce fevers voluntarily, they had no alternative under school regulations but to send him home. Body temperature can be brought under voluntary control by autonomic feedback techniques or by practice at meditation (including the daydreaming variety).

9. Where to Go from Here

WE ARE LIVING in the midst of a revolution in consciousness that will transform human society.

I cannot predict the exact nature of the change but suspect it will be a shift from straight to deep thinking on a grand scale. If external reality is the sum total of the ways people conceive of it, then external reality must change when the dominant view of it changes. Lunar consciousness is spreading through our population like a chain reaction; it cannot be stopped. And at some critical point, most of us will be experiencing our perceptions in a deep way all of the time. What will happen to external reality at that point is anybody's guess.

Joseph Wood Krutch, the humanist, wrote in 1953:

That debate which was staged during the second half of the nineteenth century between the mechanists and the humanists, between the determinists and the believers in some minimal freedom for the human being, was lost and won because of the egregious tactical error which the humanists made when they permitted the issue to depend on the existence of the "soul," instead of, as it might well have been made to depend, on the existence of consciousness. The tactical error was fatal, not merely or even chiefly because the concept of the "soul" was so closely identified with theological dogma and associated with mythologies which science really could expose as such. More important is the fact that whereas the soul is difficult to define, much less to demonstrate, "consciousness" is self-evident and yet as difficult to reconcile with complete mechanism as the soul itself.

Tactically, the error thus consisted in resting the case on the maximum rather than the minimum requirements of the debate. It permitted the chemist to say, "I cannot find the soul in my test tube," without exposing clearly the fallacy of his argument. If he had been compelled to say instead, "I cannot find consciousness in my test tube," the reply would be simple: "I don't care whether you can find it there or not. I can find it in my head. Chemistry, by failing to find it, demonstrates nothing except the limitations of its methods. I am conscious . . . and I shall continue to believe that the difference between me and a mechanism is probably very significant; even perhaps that what I find in that consciousness is better evidence concerning things to which consciousness is relevant than the things which you find in a test tube."[1]

At last we can state the terms of the debate correctly. The issue is consciousness, which is the most obvious, immediate, powerful example of nonmaterial reality as well as something all of us carry around in our heads.

The drug subculture has always been interested in consciousness. It has also always existed in this country. But never before has it included so many intelligent, "rational," ordinary, middle-class people. It is this shift of membership that has made us (that is, the thinking, rational middle class — the people who formulate conceptions of society) suddenly aware of drugs and, through them, of consciousness. Personally, I find the meaning of this phenomenon cause for great optimism.

The eruption of drugs into the rational, middle-class world is a social analog of the breaking through of nonordinary experience into an individual's ordinary awareness. It represents, above all, the tendency of the universe to reach equilibrium and harmony by balancing forces against their opposites. In *The King and the Corpse*, Heinrich Zimmer writes: " . . . every lack of integration in the human sphere simply asks for the appearance, somewhere in space and time, of the missing opposite. And the personification, the embodiment, of that predestined antagonist will inevitably show its face." The antagonistic outward appearance of drugs in America conceals a force, which is, for us, the missing opposite. It is nothing other than the reality and power of the nonmaterial, the nonrational, and the nonordinary, which we have denied for so long, and by wearing the mask it does, it compels us to take it into account, to integrate it into our conscious conceptions.

And how perfect that this force first showed its strength in the very centers of our unbalanced rationality — our universities! Why else did Alpert and Leary, representing an opposite extreme, materialize at Harvard University in 1960, except in response to a universal law by which all forces must add up to zero at any moment. This ultimate conservation law is beautifully represented by the Chinese symbol of *yin* and *yang*, which shows that the germ of the light force develops at the very heart of the dark force and vice versa, maintaining an eternal, dynamic, antagonistic equilibrium.

When we finally confront the antagonistic force that drugs symbolize in our lives and in our country, when, instead of running away from it, we let it interact with us, balance will be restored and our society will be on the way to wholeness and health. There can be no other outcome because things tend to go in one direction only — always toward equilibrium, balance, and harmony. As the power of the nonordinary gathers momentum, it will sweep us toward that equilibrium no matter what we do in our attempts to modify it. And one day, when the change has occurred, we will no doubt look back on our drug problem as something to laugh about and shake our heads over: how could we not have seen what it was really all about?

ACKNOWLEDGMENTS

AFTERWORD

WORKS CITED

SUGGESTED READING

INDEX

Acknowledgments

A number of people have helped me, both consciously and unconsciously, to write this book. I am indebted, first, to several persons who have stood by me as I have gone through the experiences that enabled me to formulate these theories and who have helped me maintain my independence from traditional intellectual forms and institutions. Conspicuous among them are my parents, my good friend Norman Zinberg, Dr. Robert Ebert of Harvard Medical School, John Kaplan of Stanford Law School, Dr. Richard Evans Schultes of the Harvard Botanical Museum, and two excellent lawyers, Neil Chayet and Brendan Sullivan.

I am also grateful to several teachers who influenced my thinking on many topics covered in this book, particularly Dr. James Gordon of the University of Pennsylvania; the late Dr. Lois Hartley, formerly of Boston College; Dr. Herbert Spiegel of the Columbia University College of Physicians and Surgeons; Dr. Phyllis Kempner of the Mount Zion Hospital Department of Psychiatry, San Francisco; and, again, Drs. Norman Zinberg and Richard Schultes.

I have received helpful suggestions from other persons who read the manuscript in its preparatory stages, among them: Richard and Anne Cotton, Winifred Rosen, Bernard Beitman, Dorothy Zinberg, Jeffrey Steingarten, Richard Stone, and Josiah Lee Auspitz. Richard Nolte of the Institute of Current World Affairs in New York City brought to my attention with uncanny timeliness writings in other fields that were highly pertinent to ideas I was developing in the manuscript. I must also thank Drs. Reese Jones, Stanley Yolles, and Tamarath Yolles, without whose collaborative efforts I would never have come to see things in this way. Finally, I must acknowledge the steady support I have received from the editors at Houghton Mifflin, particularly from Anne Barrett, who waited nearly seven years for me to be ready to write this book and who was not in the least upset that a book originally conceived as an argument for the chemical basis of mental events turned out to be an argument for the mental basis of chemical events.

ANDREW WEIL

Sterling, Virginia
Autumnal Equinox, 1971

Lee Hunsucker helped me revise this book for the 2004 new edition, identifying dated material and references and making the text more accessible to a new generation of readers.

A. W.

Afterword

After its completion, the manuscript of *The Natural Mind* was read by several distinguished members of the medical and psychiatric professions. These readers raised certain questions that will doubtless occur to others; I would like to answer them briefly.

Isn't your attack on allopathic medicine too sweeping?

Possibly. What I say is that certain basic assumptions made by orthodox physicians about the causes of disease seem to me to be unhelpful in that they do not give us much power to change disease for the better. I am not attacking the concept of healing or the ideal of a fraternity of healers. But because my questions are directed at the theoretical foundation of allopathic practice, they are necessarily a sweeping criticism. Perhaps some doctors who have read the manuscript feel that I overstate my case. If so, I have two replies. First, my own proximity to my medical education makes it hard for me to be as emotionally detached from this subject as from others; possibly five years from now I will be more moderate in my tone. Second, the case seems to me to need overstatement at this time, particularly by someone trained in allopathic methods. I say this because the power of contemporary orthodox medicine is great, and in the face of its material strength, few people without such training are able to recognize the nonmaterial weaknesses of the system and the necessity to be independent of it. Let me direct attention again to what I wrote in the text: "I do not expect readers who are allopathic practitioners or patients to accept my view on faith any more than I expect law-enforcement agents or committed drug users to accept without proof my earlier views about the dangers of drugs. But I do ask all readers to give these arguments thought and to test them against their own experience."

For a thorough critical analysis of allopathic medicine see *Health and Healing*, chapters 8–10. All of my recent work has been directed toward creating a new field of Integrative Medicine and training a new generation of physicians in mind/body interactions as well as other subjects omitted from conventional medical education. For more information, go to the Web site of the Program in Integrative Medicine of the University of Arizona: www .integrativemedicine.arizona.edu and to my own Web site: www .drweil.com.

At a certain point in life everyone dies. Maybe some of us die prematurely because we are all strung out and uptight. But maybe some yogis die for that reason, too. And maybe some yogis live to be ninety — not because of any inner peace they have found but because they haven't fallen prey to certain diseases the causes of which no one understands.

It is a common misconception among doctors that the goal of medicine is to abolish death by eliminating one by one the supposed physical causes of death. Death is a part of life; it cannot be separated from life. And if it is accepted as part of life, it is not inconsistent with the possibility of health or the healing of disease. I do not know a great deal about the longevity of yogis, but I am skeptical of longevity per se as a criterion of health. All the yogis I have met have been in good health. I have also read accounts of the deaths of some illustrious yogis and Zen masters that are much more uplifting than any deaths I have seen in the course of my experience with allopathic patients (who, when they die, are usually unconscious).

It is true that no one understands the causes of anything in an absolute sense (see chapter 1). But a major point of this book is that reality as we experience it is a product of our conceptual models and that we are free to choose among various conceptual models and that we are free to choose among various conceptual models available to us. I believe that the allopathic model with all of its assumptions (including the idea that diseases of unknown, external, material causes prey upon us) is less useful in practical terms than other available models.

Is it really possible to withdraw heroin addicts without strong medications? Heroin withdrawal can be serious.

Yes, it is possible. I have seen it happen. It may not happen very often. What interests me is that it happens sometimes because it is a very cheering piece of empirical evidence to use in developing a theory of heroin addiction. Its importance is in its demonstration that opiate withdrawal is markedly influenced by nonpharmacological factors. I do not doubt that many physicians have seen severe stomach cramps or other symptoms in withdrawing patients. But, some physicians have seen minimal physical symptoms in other patients. By paying attention to the latter cases we can become more confident in our ability to help people disengage themselves from harmful uses of narcotics without making them more dependent on material solutions to their problems.

Moreover, the observation I report will not be a surprise to physicians who have extensive experience with contemporary addicts. Some doctors have suggested that heroin today is much less potent than heroin of, say, forty years ago, and this may be a factor in the declining frequency of severe withdrawal reactions. In any case, heroin withdrawal today can be managed without strong medications, and I am strongly in favor of trying to manage it that way.

A major piece of evidence offered in support of an innate need to alter consciousness periodically is the "universality" of such methods as whirling and choking among young children. Are these practices really so universal? Or have your personal preoccupations with these practices led you to notice something that is not really typical?

I readily concede that motivation determines perception and that my preoccupations with alteration of consciousness have led me to notice these activities of children, just as preoccupations of Freudians may lead them to ignore these activities and notice other things. In much the same way, users of drugs tend to see everyone around them using drugs, while nonusers often see no one using drugs — a pattern that makes suspect all surveys to determine extent of drug use. In support of my thesis, I can only say that I have seen a great many children do these things, and that whenever I have discussed the idea with groups of adolescents, I have had no problem getting them to admit to such practices when they were younger. I have met some adults who have never heard of children spinning into dizziness or being choked by other youngsters, but I am inclined to think that they have genuinely forgotten the experiences or that they are in a minority. Anyone who wishes to assure himself of the reality of this drive should simply question children sympathetically or watch them patiently and unobtrusively when they are at play.

In saying that general anesthesia is not a pharmacological problem, you appear to disregard certain facts: that sufficient ether renders a person unconscious, that an overdose of ether kills, and that animals can be put into the anesthetic state with the drug.

I do not deny the physical reality of the effects of ether on the brain; it is a powerful depressant that interferes with consciousness. But, general anesthesia is not synonymous with unconsciousness and can be obtained with less and less of this depressant effect and greater retention of awareness the more we come to realize that it is a natural capacity of the nervous system that does not require a drug to trigger it. General anesthesia *is* a problem to pharmacologists because they cannot account for its physiological basis. It is not a problem when looked on as an altered state of consciousness.

*   *   *

I hope these comments answer some of the common questions that may be raised by medical professionals.

ANDREW WEIL

Tepoztlan, Morelos
Mexico
January 1972

Works Cited

1. What This Book Is About

1. A. T. Weil, "The Strange Case of the Harvard Drug Scandal," *Look* 27:22 (5 November 1963), p. 46.
2. Sir Humphry Davy, *Researches, Chemical and Philosophical, Chiefly Concerning Nitrous Oxide, or Dephlogisticated Nitrous Air, and Its Respiration*, London: 1839. (Accounts of experiments performed in 1799.)

2. Why People Take Drugs

1. Aldous Huxley, *The Doors of Perception* (New York: Perennial Library, 1970), pp. 9–10.
2. Huxley, p. 14.
3. Huxley, pp. 62–63.
4. D. T. Suzuki, Introduction to *Zen in the Art of Archery* by Eugen Herrigel (New York: Vintage Books, 1971), p. 10.
5. Matthew 16:26; compare Luke 10:24.
6. Patanjali, *Yoga Aphorisms* III:3, quoted by James Hewitt in *A Practical Guide to Yoga* (New York: Funk & Wagnalls, 1968), p. 146. Further commentary on this aphorism may be found in *How to Know God: The Yoga Aphorisms of Patanjali*, translated by Swami Prabhavananda and Christopher Isherwood (New York: Signet Books, 1969), pp. 122–23.

3. Is Anything Wrong with It?

1. M. M. Cohen, K. Hirshhorn, and W. A. Frosch, "In Vivo and in Vitro Chromosomal Damage Induced by LSD-25," *New England Journal of Medicine* 227 (1967), p. 1043.
2. J. H. Tjio, W. N. Pahnke, and A. A. Kurland, "LSD and Chromosomes: A Controlled Experiment," *Journal of the American Medical Association* 210 (1969), p. 849. For a review of the whole field, see N. I. Dishotsky, W. D. Loughman, R. E. Mogar, and W. R. Lipscomb, "LSD and Genetic Damage," *Science* 172 (30 April 1971), p. 431.
3. Donald G. McNeil, "Research on Ecstasy Is Clouded by Errors," *New York Times*, 2 December 2003, p. F-1.

4. Howard S. Becker, "History, Culture, and Subjective Experience: An Exploration of the Social Bases of Drug-Induced Experiences," *Journal of Health and Social Behavior* 8:3 (1967), p. 163.
5. Jerome Lettvin, "You Can't Even Step in the Same River Once," *Natural History* 76:6 (October 1967); reprinted by NIMH in *Drug Dependence* No. 2 (December 1969), p. 11.
6. Patanjali, *Yoga Aphorisms* IV:i.

4. What No One Wants to Know About Marijuana

1. A. T. Weil and N. E. Zinberg, "Acute Effects of Marijuana on Speech," *Nature* 222 (3 May 1969), p. 436.
2. Stanley F. Yolles, testimony before the Subcommittee on Public Health and Welfare of the House Interstate and Foreign Commerce Committee on H. R. 11701 and H. R. 13743 (4 February 1970).
3. Hewitt, pp. 153–54.
4. C. S. Lewis, *The Screwtape Letters* (New York: Macmillan, 1970), pp. 67–68.
5. Christmas Humphreys, *Concentration and Meditation* (Baltimore: Pelican Books, 1970), p. 36.
6. Ganga Sahai, *Metaphysical Approach to Reality* (New Delhi: Sagar Publications, 1969), pp. 50–51.
7. A. T. Weil, "Cannabis," *Science Journal* 5A:3 (September 1969), p. 41.
8. Lewis, p. 172. (The line is from an added piece, "Screwtape Proposes a Toast.")

5. Clues from the Amazon

1. Richard Evans Schultes, "Hallucinogenic Plants of the New World," *Harvard Review* 1:4 (1963), pp. 19, 20.
2. Richard Evans Schultes and Bo Holmstedt, "The Vegetal Ingredients of the Myristicaceous Snuffs of the Northwest Amazon," *Rhodora* 70 (1968), p. 781.
3. F. Brace Lamb, *Wizard of the Upper Amazon: The Story of Manuel Córdova-Rios* (Boston: Houghton Mifflin, 1974), pp. 32–33.
4. Richard Evans Schultes, "The Place of Ethnobotany in the Ethnopharmacologic Search for Psychotomimetic Drugs," in *Ethnopharmacologic Search for Psychoactive Drugs*, edited by D. H. Efron, B. Holmstedt, and N. S. Kline (NIMH-Public Health Service Publication No. 1645, 1967), p. 36.

6. The Solar Mind: Straight Thinking

1. Thomas R. Blackburn, "Sensuous-Intellectual Complementarity in Science," *Science* 172 (4 June 1971), p. 1003.

2. Humphreys, p. 83.
3. Carlos Castaneda, *The Teachings of Don Juan: A Yaqui Way of Knowledge* (New York: Ballantine Books, 1969), pp. 127–32.
4. Hewitt, p. 114.
5. *Bhagavad-Gita*, translated by Swami Prabhavananda and Christopher Isherwood (New York: Mentor Books, 1944), p. 42.
6. E. Jawetz, J. L. Melnick, and E. A. Adelberg, *Review of Medical Microbiology*, 6th ed. (Los Altos, California: Lange, 1964), p. 134.

7. A Trip to the Moon: Deep Thinking

1. Heinrich Zimmer, *The King and the Corpse*, 2d ed., edited by Joseph Campbell, Bollingen Series XI (Princeton, New Jersey: Princeton University Press, 1956), pp. 34–35.
2. Blackburn, p. 1003.
3. Lao Tzu, *The Way of Life*, translated by Witter Bynner (New York: Capricorn Books, 1962), p. 42 (verse 28).
4. *Bhagavad-Gita*, p. 36.
5. Lama Anagarika Govinda, *Foundations of Tibetan Mysticism* (New York: Samuel Weiser, Inc., 1970), p. 152.
6. From *Vigyan Bhairava* and *Sochanda Tantra*, transcribed by Paul Repa as "Centering" in *Zen Flesh, Zen Bones* (New York: Anchor Books), p. 167.
7. Lamb, pp. 156–59.
8. Lama Anagarika Govinda, *The Way of the White Clouds* (Berkeley, California: Shambala Publications, 1970), pp. 69–70.
9. William Irwin Thompson, "Beyond Contemporary Consciousness I and II," *New York Times* editorial pages, 10 May and 11 May 1971.

8. The Only Solution to the Drug Problem

1. Jay W. Forrester, "Counterintuitive Behavior of Social Systems," *Technology Review* 73:3, January 1971 (based on testimony of Professor Forrester before the Subcommittee on Urban Growth of the Committee on Banking and Currency, U.S. House of Representatives, 7 October 1970).
2. *Bhagavad-Gita*, p. 42.
3. Forrester, *op. cit.*

9. Where to Go from Here

1. Joseph Wood Krutch, *The Measure of Man* (New York: Grosset and Dunlap, 1953), pp. 120–21.

Suggested Reading

Edwin A. Abbott, *Flatland*, 5th revised ed. (New York: Barnes and Noble, 1963).

Lama Anagarika Govinda, *The Way of the White Clouds* (Berkeley, California: Shambala Publications, 1970).

James Hewitt, *A Practical Guide to Yoga* (New York: Funk & Wagnalls, 1968).

Christmas Humphreys, *Concentration and Meditation* (Baltimore: Pelican Books, 1970).

F. Bruce Lamb, *Wizard of the Upper Amazon: The Story of Manuel Córdova-Rios* (Boston: Houghton Mifflin, 1974).

Doris Lessing, *Briefing for a Descent into Hell* (New York: Alfred A. Knopf, 1971).

How to Know God: The Yoga Aphorisms of Patanjali, translated by Swami Prabhavananda and Christopher Isherwood (New York: Signet Books, 1969).

Andrew Weil, *Health and Healing: The Philosophy of Integrative Medicine and Optimum Health* (Boston: Houghton Mifflin, revised ed., 2004).

Andrew Weil, *The Marriage of the Sun and Moon: Dispatches from the Frontiers of Consciousness* (Boston: Houghton Mifflin, revised ed., 2004).

Andrew Weil and Winifred Rosen, *From Chocolate to Morphine: Everything You Need to Know About Mind-Altering Drugs* (Boston: Houghton Mifflin, revised ed, 2004).

Index

Active placebos, 83–84, 166n
Addiction treatments, 165, 183
Adolescents. *See* Children, alteration
    of consciousness and
Age regression, 28
Alcohol
    compared with other drugs, 35–37,
      42
    physical effects, 72–73
    rituals surrounding, 93
    social support for, 14–15, 19, 20
Allopathic medicine. *See also*
    Nonallopathic healing
    autonomic feedback control, 141–43
    inductive procedures in, 131
    as materialism, 122–25, 181
    principles, 121
    psychiatry, 55–57, 109, 126–27, 154
Amazonian Indians
    absence of drug problem, 86–87
    attitudes toward altered states of
      consciousness, 87–88, 91, 94
    availability of psychoactive plants,
      85–86
    model for beneficial drug use, 97–
      100
    ritualized drug use, 91–93
    set, in interpretation of psychedelic
      effects, 95–96
    use of drugs in natural form,
      88–91

Ambivalence
    acceptance of, in deep thinking,
      132–35, 155–56
    neurosis as negative experience of,
      155
    in potential of drugs, 169–70
Amotivation, marijuana use and, 4, 51n
Anesthesia, 28, 82, 149–51, 184
Anxiety
    psychedelic drugs use, 54
    subjective, marijuana and, 76–77
Arnold, Edwin, 59
Autonomic nervous system. *See also*
    Nonallopathic healing
    autonomic feedback control, 141–43,
      173n
    conscious control of, 28–29, 125,
      138–44

Bad trips, panic reactions to drugs,
    44–46, 136
Barbiturates, overdoses of, 37
Becker, Howard, 45–46
Benign paranoia, 155
Bhagavad-Gita, 112–13, 134–35, 166
Bias
    attitudes toward alcohol, 14
    descriptions of drug-associated
      behavior, 54–57
    divergent interpretations of data,
      4–8

Bias (*cont.*)
in scientific community, 99–100
single-blind experiments, 65–66
Weil's, 8–9, 181, 184
Biological drive to alter consciousness,
16, 31, 168
Blackburn, Thomas R., 104
Brain damage, ecstasy and, 39
Buddhism, 30, 58–59

Cannabis. *See* Marijuana
Castaneda, Carlos, 110–12
Children, alteration of consciousness
and
age at start of drug use, 51n
Amazonian Indians, 91
explorations, 16–21, 31, 168, 183–84
fear, guilt, secrecy, 17–20, 168
Chromosomal damage, LSD and, 37–
39
Coexisting opposites, 132–33
Collective consciousness
Amazonian tribal unity, 157–60
extrasensory perceptions and telepathy, 160–62
between healer and patient, 148,
160
Concentration and relaxation
control of autonomic nervous system, 139–40
sharing of consciousness, 161
Consciousness, alteration of. *See also*
Meditation
absence of physical correlates, 26–
27
Amazonian Indians, 87–88, 91, 94,
95
anesthesia as, 28, 82, 149–51, 184
confusion with drug use, 33
continuum across states of consciousness, 27–28

control of autonomic nervous system, 28–29, 138–41
correlation between psychosis and
genius, 30, 46–47
daydreaming, 27, 29, 30, 173
desirability of, 25–26, 31, 168
Eastern versus Western approaches
to, 26–27, 151–53, 172
fear, guilt, secrecy among children,
17–20, 168
Freudian analogy to sexual experience, 16, 18
as innate, normal drive, 15–20, 31,
168
intuitive flashes, 130
loss of sense of ego, 29–30
perception of sensory information,
81–83
shared, 148, 157–62
simultaneous experience of opposites, 133
Crowley, Aleister, 58–59

Davy, Humphry, 10
Daydreaming, 27, 29, 30, 173
Deductive reasoning, 132
Deep thinking. *See also* Consciousness, alteration of
acceptance of ambivalence, 132–35,
155–56, 169–70
anesthesia, 28, 82, 149–51, 184
control of autonomic nervous system, 28–29, 125, 138–44
episodic flashes, 129–30
nonallopathic healing, 144–49, 160
positive experience of infinity, 135–
37
positive neurosis and psychosis,
155–57
positive paranoia, 153–55
reliance on intuition, 129–32, 161

shared consciousness, 148, 157–62
synthesis of Eastern and Western
    approaches, 26–27, 139, 151–53,
    172
Dependence upon drugs, 35, 54–55,
    59, 88, 124
Depression and despair, 116–18
Differences, perception of, 114–16
Direct experience versus intellect,
    104–8
Disease
    allopathic medicine, 121–26, 131,
        141–43, 181
    allopathic psychiatry, 55–57, 109,
        126–27, 154
    autonomic nervous system, 28–29,
        125, 138–44
    cause of, 123–25, 144–46
    nonallopathic healing, 144–49, 160
Dole, Vincent, 165n
Drugless high, 83, 98–99
Drug problem
    addiction treatments, 165, 183
    dependence as error in thinking, 59,
        124
    drug use versus abuse, 31
    erroneous conceptual models, 9–10,
        167–68
    exacerbation of, 163–66
    means for solving, 169–73
    nature of consciousness and, 1–2
    potency of drugs, 88–89
Drug use. See also specific aspects of
        drug use
    beneficial, Indian model for, 97–
        100
    confusion with alteration of con-
        sciousness, 33
    innate drive to alter consciousness,
        15–16, 17, 19, 20, 168
    intravenous, 97–98

learning from users, 99–100, 171–
    72
natural form of drugs, 89–91, 97–
    99
negative versus positive reasons for,
    94–95, 100
progression theory, 51–52
toxicity of drug, 40
ubiquity of, 14
use versus abuse, 31
Drug use, arguments against
    false issues, 51–57
    medical
        brain damage, 39
        chromosomal damage, 37–39
        liver and nerve damage, 40
        respiratory damage, 41
        tolerance and withdrawal, 35–37
    practical, 57–62
    psychological
        dependence, 54–55
        panic reaction, 44–46
        psychosis, 46–48
        tolerance, 48–51
        toxic psychosis, 42–44, 74
Dysfunction, mental. See Mental
    health issues

Eastern approach to consciousness
    Buddhism, 30, 58–59
    emphasis on direct experience, 26–
        27, 152–53, 172
    yoga, 29–30, 58–59, 79, 139–40
Ecstasy (MDMA), 15, 39, 48, 59, 60
Ego
    development of, in children, 17–18
    sense of, in altered states of con-
        sciousness, 29–30
Ego-centered consciousness. See
    Straight thinking
Episodic flashes, 129–30

Escape. *See* Consciousness, alteration
     of
Experimental studies of marijuana.
     See also Marijuana
   in early twentieth century, 64–65
   impairment of psychological perfor-
     mance, 74–75
   influence of set and setting, 65–
     66
   negative hypotheses, 81–82
   Weil's, 66–70
Extrasensory perceptions, 157–62

Faith healing, 148–49
Fear and guilt, alteration of conscious-
     ness and, 17–20, 168
Feedback control, autonomic, 141–43
Flashbacks, 52–53
Flashes, intuitive, 130
Forrester, Jay W., 164, 167

Genius, nonordinary modes of con-
     sciousness and, 30, 46–47
Govinda, Lama Anagarika, 140, 160–
     61

Healing. *See* Allopathic medicine;
     Nonallopathic healing
Hemp drugs. *See* Marijuana
Heroin, 35–37, 49–50, 165, 183
Hewitt, James, 79
Highs, drug-induced versus drugless,
     60–61
Holmstedt, Bo, 86–87
Homeopathy, 146
Humphreys, Christmas, 80, 105
Huxley, Aldous, 22–23
Hypnosis
   analgesia, 28, 82, 149
   change of ordinary mode of con-
     sciousness, 22

control of autonomic nervous sys-
     tem, 28, 139

Illness. *See* Disease
Imagination, visual, 161–62
Immediate memory, 77–81
Immediate reality of present, 77–81,
     159
Indian model for beneficial drug use,
     97–100. *See also* Amazonian
     Indians
Infinity, positive experience of, 135–37
Intellect. *See also* Straight thinking
   abandonment of, 105–6, 159–60
   negative experience of infinity, 136–
     37
   perception of differences, 114–16
   plus intuition, in deep thinking,
     131–32
   reliance on, in straight thinking,
     104–8
Intoxication. *See* Consciousness, alter-
     ation of; Drug use
Intravenous drug use, 97–98
Intuition, 129–32, 161. *See also* Deep
     thinking

Journalism, bias in, 8–9

Knowledge. *See* Deep thinking;
     Straight thinking
Koch's Postulates, 122–23
Krishnamurti, J., 80–81
Krutch, Joseph Wood, 174–75

Lao Tzu, 134
Legal issues concerning drugs, 167–
     68
Lettvin, Jerome, 53–54
Lewis, C. S., 79–80
Limbic brain system, 144–45

LSD, 37–39, 45–46
Lunar mind. *See* Deep thinking

Marijuana
  as active placebo, 83
  amotivation, 4, 51
  classification of, 70–71
  experimental studies, Weil's, 66–70
  experimental studies in early twen-
    tieth century, 64–65
  health consequences, 40–41
  immediate memory, 77–78, 81
  ingestion of, toxic psychosis and, 74
  legalization, 167–68
  overcaution and compensation in
    performance, 75–76
  panic reaction, 45
  perceptual changes, 81–82
  physical effects, 70–73
  potency, 71
  psychological effects, 74–75, 81
  ritual surrounding, 93
  set and setting in individual re-
    sponse to, 65
  speech, 76–77
  subjective anxiety, 76, 78
  therapeutic ratio, 40
  unconscious memories, 27–28
Materialism
  in addiction treatment, 165
  in allopathic medicine, 122–25, 181
  causality attributed to external real-
    ity, 113–14
MDMA (ecstasy), 15, 39, 48, 59, 60
Medicine, allopathic. *See* Allopathic
    medicine
Meditation
  abandonment of intellect, 105
  analgesia through, 149
  change in ordinary mode of con-
    sciousness, 22

control of autonomic nervous sys-
    tem, 29, 139, 173n
  focus on immediate present reality,
    80
  highs obtainable through, 58, 59
  loss of sense of ego, 30
  sensory detachment from external
    reality, 112
  similarity to trance, 27
Memory, immediate, 77–81
Mental health issues
  allopathic view of, 55–57, 126–27,
    154
  flashbacks, 52–53
  neurosis, 155–56
  panic reactions, 45–46
  paranoia, 153–55
  psychosis, 42–44, 46–48, 56n, 74,
    156–57
Mescaline, 21–25, 25
Methadone, 61, 165
Mind. *See* Consciousness, alteration
    of; Deep thinking; Straight
    thinking

Natural form of drugs, 89–91, 97–99
Negative paranoia, 153–55
Negative psychosis, 46–48, 56n
Nervous system, autonomic. *See also*
    Nonallopathic healing
  autonomic feedback control, 141–43,
    173n
  conscious control of, 28–29, 125,
    138–44
Neurophysiology, 139–40
Neurosis, 126–27, 155–56
Nitrous oxide (laughing gas), 10, 61,
    150
Nonallopathic healing
  communication between healer and
    patient, 148, 160

Nonallopathic healing (*cont.*)
    control of autonomic nervous sys-
        tem, 28–29, 125, 138–44
    faith healing, 148–49
    role of patient, 147–48
    theoretical basis, 145–46
    unconscious mind as cause of dis-
        ease, 123–24, 144–46
Nonordinary reality. *See* Conscious-
    ness, alteration of
Nonordinary thinking. *See* Deep
    thinking
Nutmeg, 63–64, 166n

Ordinary thinking. *See* Straight
    thinking
Overdose of drugs, 37, 42–44, 74

Panic reaction to drugs, 44–46, 136
Paranoia, 153–55
Patanjali, 30, 58, 112
Pattern-forming tendency of uncon-
    scious mind, 154–55
Performance, marijuana and, 74–76
Pessimism, 116–18
Political action, 127–28
Positive neurosis, 155–56
Positive paranoia, 153–55
Positive psychosis, 156–57
Pot. *See* Marijuana
Potency of drugs, 71, 88–91
Pregnancy, drug use during, 41
Present moment, 77–81
Psilocybin, 24
Psychedelic drugs, importance of set
    and setting, 24. *See also* LSD
Psychiatry, allopathic model in, 55–57,
    109, 126–27, 154
Psychological arguments against drug
    use
    dependence, 54–55

panic reaction, 44–46
psychosis, 46–48
tolerance, 48–51
toxic psychosis, 42–44, 74
Psychosis
    definition, 46
    negative, 46–48, 56n
    positive, 156–57
    toxic psychosis, 42–44, 74
Psychosomatic nature of illness, 123–
    25, 144–46
Purity of drugs, 88–91

Reality. *See* Deep thinking; Straight
    thinking
Reality testing, 46
Relaxation and concentration, 139–40,
    141, 161
Religious systems. *See also* Yoga
    antidrug dogma, 57–59
    immediate reality of present, 78–
        81
    loss of sense of self, 30
Respiratory system, effects of mari-
    juana on, 41
Reverse tolerance, 73
Ricuarte, George A., 39
Ritual surrounding drug use, 91–94,
    99

Sahai, Ganga, 80–81
Schizophrenia, 157
Schultes, Richard Evans, 63, 86–87,
    96
Science. *See also* Allopathic medicine
    Eastern versus Western, 26–27
    flawed, 38–39
    inductive procedures in, 131
    wrongly stated hypotheses, 6–8
Secrecy concerning alteration of con-
    sciousness, 17–20, 168

Self, sense of
  in altered states of consciousness,
    29–30
  development of, in children, 17–18
Senses, attachment to, 108–13, 130–31
Set and setting
  interpretation of psychedelic effects,
    95–96
  panic reactions, 44–46
  study of drugs, 65
  variable responses to drugs, 24–25
  withdrawal from heroin, 36
Sexual experience, compared to alter-
    ation of consciousness, 15, 16,
    18
Shared consciousness
  Amazonian tribal unity, 157–60
  extrasensory perceptions and telepa-
    thy, 160–62
  between healer and patient, 148,
    160
Sleep, fear of, among children, 18
Sleep and wakefulness, transition
    between, 16–17, 153
Solar mind. See Straight thinking
Speech, effect of marijuana on, 76–
    77
Speed (drug), 48–49
Spiritual experiences
  drug use and, 57–59
  immediate reality of present, 78–81
  loss of sense of self, 30
Spontaneous high, 83, 98–99
Straight thinking
  acceptance of appearance as reality,
    113–14
  allopathic medicine, 121–26, 131,
    141–43, 181
  allopathic model in psychiatry, 55–
    57, 109, 126–27, 154

attachment to intellect, 104–8
attachment to senses, 108–13, 130–
    31
chain of false logic, 117
fear of ambivalence, 127
incomprehensibility of nonordinary
    reality, 110–12
materialism, 113–14, 122–25, 181
negative experience of infinity, 136–
    37
negativity, isolation, despair, 116–18
perception of differences, 114–16
political action, 127–28
predominance of, 103
use of insecticides and antibiotics,
    118–20
Suzuki, D. T., 30

Teenagers. See Children, alteration of
    consciousness and
Telepathic communication, 162
Therapeutic ratio of marijuana, 40
Thinking. See Deep thinking; Straight
    thinking
Tobacco, 35–36, 41–42, 49
Tolerance to drugs
  disruption of life, 48–51
  reverse tolerance, 73
  subjective tolerance, 60
  withdrawal, 35–37, 138
Toxicity of drugs, 40
Toxic psychosis, 42–44, 74
Tranquilizers, 56n
True healing. See Nonallopathic heal-
    ing
Twelve-step programs, 165–66

Unconscious mind. See Conscious-
    ness, alteration of; Deep
    thinking

Unity
  acceptance of ambivalence, 132–35,
    155–56
  among Amazonian Indians, 157–
    60
  channels between conscious and
    unconscious minds, 131, 143–
    44
  perception of similarities, 115

Visionary experience, 21–22
Visual imagination, 161–62

Withdrawal from drugs, 35–37, 183

Yoga
  antidrug dogma, 58–59

  control of autonomic nervous sys-
    tem, 29, 139–40
  as experiential science of conscious-
    ness, 26
  focus on immediate present reality,
    79
  loss of sense of ego, 30
  psychic powers available through,
    161

Zen archery, 29–30
Zimmer, Heinrich, 132–33
Zinberg, Norman, 66–70, 76–77

ABOUT THE AUTHOR

Andrew Weil, M.D., is the best-selling author of ten books, including *Spontaneous Healing, Eating Well for Optimum Health, Eight Weeks to Optimum Health,* and forthcoming, *Healthy Aging.* Dr. Weil has degrees in biology and medicine from Harvard University. He has experienced and studied healers and healing systems around the world and has earned an international reputation as an expert on alternative medicine, mind-body interactions, and medical botany. He is Clinical Professor of Medicine and director of the Program in Integrative Medicine (www.integrativemedicine.arizona.edu) at the University of Arizona in Tucson. Dr. Weil also writes a monthly newsletter, *Self Healing* (www.drweilselfhealing.com) and has a popular Web site, www.drweil.com.

NATURAL HEALTH, NATURAL MEDICINE
The Complete Guide to Wellness and Self-Care for Optimum Health

A comprehensive guide to preventative health maintenance and the foundation for Dr. Andrew Weil's work on maintaining optimum health. *Natural Health, Natural Medicine* is the bible of natural medicine, featuring general diet and nutrition information as well as simple recipes, answers to readers' most pressing questions, a catalog of home remedies, invaluable resources, and hundreds of practical tips.
ISBN 0-618-47903-1

HEALTH AND HEALING
The Philosophy of Integrative Medicine and Optimum Health

Dr. Weil's groundbreaking handbook for people who want to understand the strengths and weaknesses of conventional and alternative medicine, *Health and Healing* presents the full spectrum of alternative healing practices, including holistic medicine, homeopathy, osteopathy, chiropractic, and Chinese medicine, and outlines how they differ from conventional approaches. ISBN 0-618-47908-2

FROM CHOCOLATE TO MORPHINE
WITH WINIFRED ROSEN
Everything You Need to Know About Mind-Altering Drugs

The definitive guide to drugs and drug use, now revised and updated to cover drugs made available in the last decade. This enormously popular book is the best and most authoritative resource for unbiased information about how drugs affect the mind and the body. ISBN 0-618-48379-9

THE MARRIAGE OF THE SUN AND MOON
Dispatches from the Frontiers of Consciousness

A collection of essays about Dr. Weil's travels to South America in the early 1970s in search of information on altered states of consciousness, drug use in other cultures, and other matters having to do with the complementarity of mind and body. These experiences laid the foundation of his mission to restore the connection between medicine and nature. ISBN 0-618-47905-8

THE NATURAL MIND
A Revolutionary Approach to the Drug Problem

Dr. Weil's first book and the philosophical basis for all of his resulting beliefs and tenets on health, healing, and the mind. Now completely revised and updated for the twenty-first century, this is essential reading for anyone interested in Dr. Weil's philosophy of integrative medicine and optimum health. ISBN 0-618-46513-8

Made in the USA
Middletown, DE
23 May 2021